ERECTILE DYSFUNCTION

A GUIDE FOR PARTNERS

"I believe this is a terrific contribution and reflects a real-world patent perspective, that is not shown in books written by medical professionals. I commend Elisha for telling her and Bruce's personal story."

Reviewed by: Arthur L. Burnett II, MD, MBA, FACS
Johns Hopkins Medical Center
Internationally acclaimed urologic surgeon and
a preeminent doctor in his field.

Elisha J. Nixon Cobb, Ph.D, M.Ed.

Edited, Formatting & Cover Design by:
Ya Ya Ya Creative – www.YaYaYaCreative.com

ISBN: 978-1-7368803-4-0

PRINTED AND BOUND IN THE UNITED STATES OF AMERICA

To my late husband, Bruce J. Cobb

that you may rest in peace knowing you left a legacy of unwavering service dedicated to students, faculty, staff, and community members that will endure for generations to come.

To my late parents
my mother, Etheleen Morris
my father, Landis Morris

that your children may continue to show the kind of mercy, love, and caring that you bestowed on us and others all the days of our lives.

Preface

E xperiencing erectile dysfunction (ED) for most couples can be a time of confusion, isolation and loneliness, but the journey of finding a solution to a problem that affects a man and his partner can instead be one of clarity, partnership, and hope. In addition the decision about which treatment options are best for you and your partner's particular situation maybe a contributing factor to an already confusing time as well. What can lessen the anxiety is the unwavering support of partners who are in relationships with men experiencing erectile dysfunction. A partner's attitude, sensitivity, and understanding can have a direct effect on the man's mental and emotional state, making the help-seeking and compliance behavior a positive part of the ED experience. Therefore, it's critical that clinicians encourage both partners to be included during all phases of the journey to finding an ideal solution to erectile dysfunction.

This book provides personal insights about how my husband and I coped with erectile dysfunction along with the day-to-day challenges, decisions, and lessons learned as we sought a solution to his erection problem. In addition, the chapter of the book highlighting the comments and opinions of eleven African American men about their partner's role will offer additional support for you and your partner. Hopefully, you and your partner will find our journey and the comments from men who volunteered to be a part of this book enlightening and empowering—enough to ease any doubts or feelings of being confused or alone. I applaud you both for making the decision to partner with each other and with your medical professionals in seeking the best care possible to succeed.

Acknowledgments

A debt of gratitude is owed to my daughter Marcella L. Nixon for her support and encouragement in the completion of this book. Her inspiration and guidance have been a beacon of light from start to finish. Next, my two sons Patrick and Jeffrey, for the joys of seeing them transform from boys to men and whose moral and intellectual insights have cheered me on through my darkest moments.

My deepest gratitude I extend to Arthur L. Burnett, II, MD, MBA, FACS, who I have come to know with kindness as Bud Burnett. He has been a bulwark of strength, encouragement, and unwavering support to Bruce and me throughout our journey. His expertise and generous ability to show empathy and caring made a confusing stretch of time dealing with erectile dysfunction more comprehensible, and hopeful. In preparing this book, I drew on many of his outstanding publications. I am thankful for his medical insights and support in his review of the initial draft of this book.

Many thanks go to the eleven men whose personal perspectives on the role of the partner who is in a relationship with a man dealing with men with erectile dysfunction added to the richness of this book.

With much appreciation, I feel obligated to mention their anonymous names: B.J., Caleb LV, C-Low, Fred, J.R., Jesse, Joe, Luke, Markus, Steve, and Nate.

Many others whose confidence in me have enriched my personal and professional growth down through the years. They include Collins O. Airhihenbuwa, PhD, MPH, my graduate professor and mentor. His teaching and writing style have been an inspiration in writing this book. As his student, I have learned much about the effect culture has in determining perceptions and treatment options. Others include Bruce's son, Brandon for his feedback in the preparation of this book. Louis G. whose prayers and unwavering support have served to bolster my confidence in completing this book. Gwenny, my dear friend, my younger sister, Denise, and my brothers Kim and Landis, all of whom are my greatest cheerleaders. Their encouragement is unbounding.

Finally, I would like to thank my editor, Barbara Rodriguez and her assistants, and publishers at Unplugged Publications, Bishop R. C. Blakes, Jr and his wife Lisa for their support in the final publication of this book.

Introduction

How To Use This Book To Benefit You and Your Partner

Oh, he's just slowing down because he's older, so I thought at first. Other than aging, my 66-year-old partner and I didn't have a clue as to what was happening. All we knew was that our sex life was changing as a result of my husband having problems achieving an erection. He was confused, and so was I. What added to our confusion was that we didn't know where to turn, or how to talk about *it*, a word my partner and I conveniently used to describe his inability to achieve an erection. Our discovering a way to openly and honestly talk about *it*, enabled us to work together to find a solution to the problem.

This book is a beginner's guide to helping singles and couples understand their respective roles in finding a solution to a problem that affects both partners. This book will help you understand some of the symptoms, causes, and available treatment options that can help you and your partner map out a plan of action so that you both can once again enjoy a satisfying sexual experience and quality of life you deserve. Included are how-to-cope strategies related to improving communication with your partner, self-care, and preparing for a doctor's visit, or an overnight hospital stay for surgery.

This book is broken down into chapters, followed by references, a list of credible organizations, books for further reading, a glossary used in relationship to erectile dysfunction, and an index. I am confident that you and your partner will find this information useful in making the right decision for your given situation. So let's start by creating an atmosphere where you both can begin to talk freely about the *it* in the room.

Table of Contents

What is Erectile Dysfunction?
Knowing When It's Time to Talk, Let Pain Points Lead the Way.
How to Create a Safe Place to Begin the Conversation.
Tips to Help Couples Tackle Erectile Dysfunction Together.
The Stigma of Loss of Manhood in Men with Sexual Dysfunction.
When Your Partner is Reluctant to Talk About HIs Erectile Dysfunction.
Why is Self-Care Important?

The Internal and External Organs of Male Reproductive Anatomy.
It's Smaller Than It Appears.

Sexual Drive and Libido Phase.
Sexual Arousal and Erection Phase.
Orgasm and Ejaculation Phase.

When Blood Flow Is Interrupted: Causes and Risk Factors.
Knowing When to Seek Help.

Finding a Solution for Erectile Dysfunction.
Non-Invasive First Line Treatment Options.
Invasive Treatment Options Requiring Surgery.

CHAPTER 1

Creating a Safe Place For Partners to Communicate

Babe, I'm Sorry. It's not working...

This wasn't the first time that *it* happened. *It* happened several times prior, and still we could not talk about *it*. The *it* that we were reluctant to talk about is called erectile dysfunction (ED). We both heard of the term, but neither one of us knew what the term meant, nor did we know what to do about it.

Erectile dysfunction is defined as the persistent inability to achieve or maintain penile erection sufficient for satisfactory sexual performance. The key word here is 'persistent.' It is normal for some men to have occasional trouble getting or keeping an erection, but if the problem becomes frequent or lasts a long time, it's an issue that requires medical attention.

Not having sexual intercourse on a regular basis really wasn't a concern at first until we both started avoiding sexual intimacy by making excuses like "I'm really tired" or 'We better get some rest because we got to get up early in the morning." I was also going to bed earlier than usual. Sometimes he would retire first then I would follow much later. It was then I realized that avoiding the issue can't go on. Our silence was not helping at all. The fact was that erectile dysfunction was affecting our sex lives and enjoyable time spent together just talking about everything, yet nothing at all. Erectile dysfunction was surely having a significant impact on my husband's quality of life and mine.

Knowing When It's Time to Talk, Let Pain Points Lead the Way

We needed to talk, but I didn't know where to begin. How do couples begin to talk about erectile dysfunction, a taboo issue that has so many *stigmas* that can affect a man's self-esteem? One thing I didn't want to do if I brought the subject up was to add his discomfort, but I knew if we were ever going to find a solution, we had to start talking. So I thought I would try to break the routine of coming home from work, eating, and making small talk by asking him how he was feeling about our not being sexually active. A risky question, for sure. When he immediately got up to pour another glass of wine, I could tell he was a bit edgy and somewhat taken aback by the question just as I was taken aback by his response. When he returned, he finally opened up and said,

> I don't know how I feel at times. Sometimes, I guess I'm not in the mood for sex. Other times when I am in the mood, babe it's just not working. I don't want to let you down, so I just don't think about trying anything at all. I don't know why I'm having erections during the day, it's embarrassing. I don't know what's happening.

His willingness to share his feeling motivated me to create a safe place to continue our talks without blame or embarrassment. Knowing when it's the right time to talk about ED with a partner affected by ED is not easy to determine. For us, the right time to discuss ED evolved from our being isolated and feeing alone, especially in the evening. My advice is to start with his pain points.

A pain point is a problem, obstacle, or complication that causes discomfort. Pain point examples related to the inability to achieve or maintain erection include fear of seeing a doctor, lack of knowledge about what's happening physically and emotionally, a non-supportive partner, or a partner's negative reaction to a man's inability to achieve an erection. A good place to start is to listen closely to what your partner is saying about himself, or his condition. What he says could about how he is feeling could very well be a pain point that opens the door to an intimate moment of sharing. Here are some tips that I found helpful in creating a safe place for sharing.

How to Create a Safe Place to Begin the Conversation

1. Express your feelings first then allow your partner to express his—with no interruptions. Listening is a skill, it is something that is learned. So begin to practice now since the journey to finding a solution to your partner's erectile issue will definitely present additional opportunities in which listening is a critical part of being supportive.

2. Do not make assumptions because you really may not know what your husband feels as a man. Let him tell you what he is feeling.

3. Remind him that he is not alone, and that you are all in for the long haul. No matter what.

4. Keep confidentiality. What you and your partner share should stay between you and your partner. For him to speak freely, he must feel safe even if you don't understand fully what he may be experiencing emotionally or physically. Keeping confidentiality means the listening partner has to deny self. Once again, do not interrupt or interject your own feelings no matter how valid. Allow for your mate to empty himself or complete his sharing about what he is experiencing physically and emotionally.

5. Offer to go to the doctor with him when the time comes. He may want to go alone, but at least he knows you want to be there.

When he is ready to talk further, here are some tips to help couples to continue tackling ED together.

Tips To Help Couples Tackle Erectile Dysfunction Together

1. Don't ignore the issue, not only won't it go away, it is actually likely to worsen.

2. Take the problem out of the bedroom when you find time to talk.

3. Don't rush in and blurt things without thinking about what you are both going to say to each other and the consequences of those words.

4. It's important to medicalize the problem by referring to it as ED rather than using words like it or impotence, both of which carry a negative connotation of denial or blame.

5. Talking about erectile dysfunction is one thing, the next step is tackling it. If you make progress in discussions, the next step is to make an action plan. If at first you don't succeed don't assume this means failure, it just means you haven't yet reached a solution.

6. Remember the importance of romantic actions and gestures. Something as simple as a peck on the cheek or arm round the shoulder reinforces your bond when you feel that you might be drifting apart.

7. Be honest with each other. Speaking about ED is the time to lay your cards on the table and talk frankly about how life is going; stress and depression can be big players where ED is concerned, as can drugs and alcohol.

8. Do some background reading on ED. In your conversations, the affected partner may recognize that the presenting problem represents far more than not being able to perform. Erectile dysfunction could be the symptoms of an underlying issue so don't dismiss it.

9. Interact with a health care professional face-to-face or online to find out what treatments are available.[1]

But what if your partner is reluctant to share? Feeling embarrassed and ashamed about health problems may prevent many men from talking about their sexual health with their partner.

The Stigma of Loss of Manhood in Men With Sexual Dysfunction

The stigmas associated with a man's inability to perform sexually are many. The loss of manhood and lack of masculinity are two of the biggest issues in terms of stigma. Even going to see a clinician to discuss treatment carries a stigma. Anticipating seeing a same sex urologist let alone having the urologist perform a digital rectal exam by inserting a finger into a man's rectum to feel for nodules in the back of prostate gland is not only somewhat painful for men, the procedure can also leave them men feeling resentful and violated.

Other stigmas are related to treatment and therapy. Some men who have been socialized to be strong may feel they do not need therapy or medication. Surgeons who deal with sexual medicine have many patients who want to keep things quiet, sometimes with their partners or even exploring male health clinics without telling their regular physicians.[2]

Unless both partners are willing to engage in open and honest communication, any discussion about sex may trigger feelings of guilt, anger, blame, or embarrassment, setting back rather than moving forward to a solution. Here are some suggestions to help your partner to cope with his reluctance to communicate.

When Your Partner With ED Is Reluctant To Talk About His Erectile Dysfunction

1. As his partner, gently attempt to take charge, which is not the same as taking control. Taking charge of a situation can lead the way to you both taking ownership of the problem as a couple. By

taking the lead—and suggesting couples counseling, if needed— you can bring the issue into the light and use the process to strengthen, rather than hurt, the relationship.

2. If your partner doesn't know what is causing the problem but acknowledges its existence, suggest a physical exam with the urologist.

3. Make every effort to express yourself with sensitivity and without any suggestion of blame. While it is important to share your worries, do so within the context of the relationship rather than asserting how "you" are causing "me" to worry. That is where worry turns to blame.[3]

Needless to say, experiencing erectile dysfunction is not something a man should go through alone, even though many do. But if you are in partnership with a man whose dealing with erectile dysfunction, it is important that you take care of your mental health while supporting your partner.

Self-care:
Ways to Take Care of Your Mental Health While Supporting Your Partner During a Stretch of Erectile Dysfunction

1. Carve out alone time. Both partners need it to maintain a healthy relationship.

2. Step away from the issue at times. You don't want to live in a state of depression, worry, or hopelessness. Life offers much more than sex. Find ways to make you happy.

3. Stay clear of any codependent tendencies on his part. Some men may obsess over the psychological trauma of experiencing erectile dysfunction by keep referring to themselves as being less than a man, making the problem worse. You are there to support him, not to own his problem or feel responsible for his condition.

4. Don't permit his ED to take all of your time. The same advice in #3 goes for you, do not obsess over the issue yourself, it's unfair if he keeps you trapped in his own thoughts.

5. Have a plan when obsessive conversations persist. Be direct, but kindly state that you need to take a walk or change the subject by reminding him that his feelings do not take away from your commitment to him. If boundaries become an issue, don't be afraid to seek counseling or spiritual help for yourself as this will help both of you.

Regardless of whether your partner is ready to talk or not, a plan of action is needed. If he is unwilling to talk about erectile dysfunction, give him more time, but continue to take care of you while gathering more information that will help you to better understand erectile dysfunction.[4]

Learning the basic structure and function of the male reproduction anatomy might be a good place to start.

CHAPTER 2

The Male Reproductive Anatomy

Nobody's penis is that big.

T he *penis* is an amazing organ that serves many functions. The penis functions as a reproductive organ. The penis functions as an organ for urination as well as an organ for intimacy and sexual relations. To understand how an erection occurs, it probably best to start with understanding the male reproductive anatomy. In **Figure 1** (below), the shaft and shape of the penis resembles a cucumber.

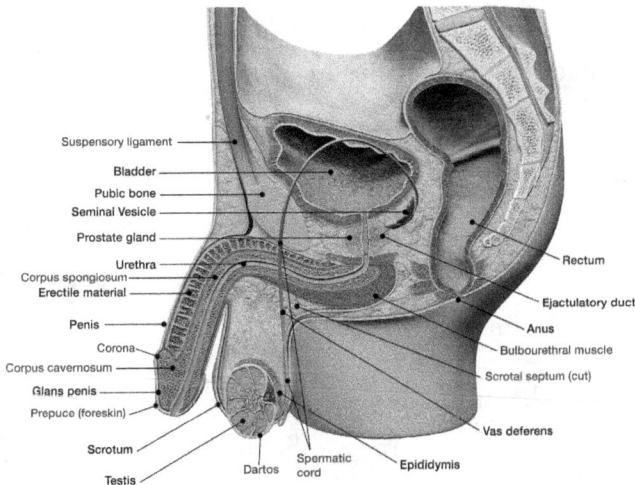

Figure 1: *Penis | Description, Anatomy, & Physiology*

The shaft or what one sees externally is not actually the full size of the penis. An internal part of the penis, the part that is not visible, connects to the pelvic bones inside the body. Situated on the outside of the penis is another organ: the scrotum. The role of the scrotum is to protect the testes and maintain a temperature vital to the production of sperm and testosterone, a hormone not only responsible for male secondary sexual characteristics such as facial and body hair, pelvic build (not rounded hips characteristic of women's hips), upper body masculine build, ability to generate muscle mass at a rate faster than women, and penile function, which is the main focus of this book.[1]

The head or tip of the penis biologically referred to as the *glans*. Inside the penis is a tube called the *urethra* that passes through the center releases both semen from the ejaculatory ducts (located on each side of the *prostate gland*) delivers sperm into the urethra. The urethra also expels semen from the prostate (located just below the bladder in front of the rectum), and the seminal vesicles (located behind the bladder but in front of the rectum) and urine from the *bladder*. It might seem that semen and urine are expelled at the same time from the urethra. The amazing thing about the internal structure of the penis is that there is a valve like organ called the sphincter muscle located near the neck of the bladder that helps hold urine until a man is ready to urinate. During orgasm, that same muscle contracts to keep ejaculate from entering the bladder.[1]

In addition to the urethra, there are three additional tubes worth mentioning: two corpora cavernosa tubes located side by side and one corpus spongiosum located midway beneath the *corpus spongiosum*. **Figure 2** (page 11), shows the tissue inside the penis that's responsible for facilitating erections, the corpora cavernosum. This mass of spongy-like tissue fills with blood like a sponge. The corpora cavernosum is surrounded by muscles that support the penis when erect and during ejaculation.

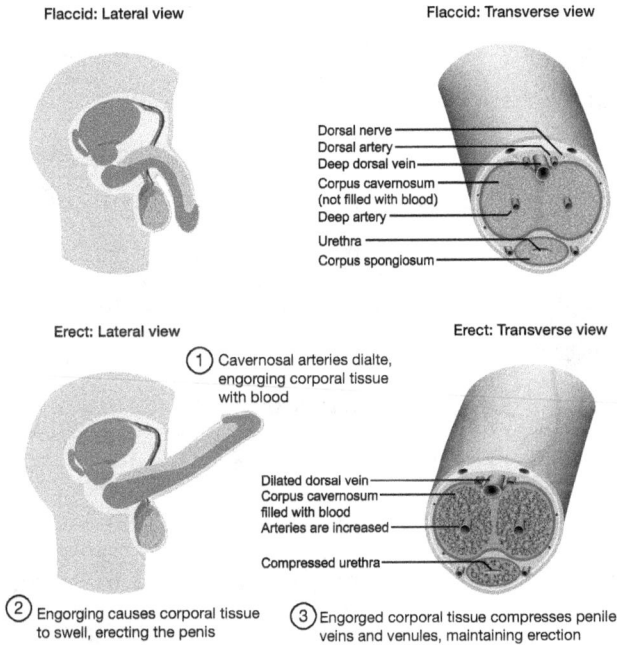

Flaccid: Lateral view

Flaccid: Transverse view

Dorsal nerve
Dorsal artery
Deep dorsal vein
Corpus cavernosum
(not filled with blood)
Deep artery
Urethra
Corpus spongiosum

Erect: Lateral view

Erect: Transverse view

① Cavernosal arteries dialte, engorging corporal tissue with blood

Dilated dorsal vein
Corpus cavernosum
filled with blood
Arteries are increased
Compressed urethra

② Engorging causes corporal tissue to swell, erecting the penis

③ Engorged corporal tissue compresses penile veins and venules, maintaining erection

Figure 2: *Cross-Sectional Anatmy of Penis.*

When filled with blood, the penis goes from flaccid (limp) to erect (stiff). Together all three organs are situated similar to the shape of a triangle. It's the spongy texture of corpora cavernosa and corpus spongiosum that becomes engorged with blood that causes an erection. All three organs consist of smooth muscle cells, nerves, tiny cells that line the inside of blood vessels, and fibers that allow the lengthening and increase of the penile stiffness during erection, as well as the rapid return to a flaccid state after sexual arousal.[1]

It's Smaller Than It Appears

The idea of you and your partner looking at a drawing of a penis may be a bit unrealistic or even strange. It could actually be a time of relaxation that diverts attention away from thinking about dysfunction. Bruce truly had a sense of humor about almost everything. In fun, Bruce drew a picture of a penis that was about 8 inches long. All I could say in response was...*really.* The average length of an erect penis is between 5.1 inches and 5.5 inches. The average length of a flaccid (limp) penis 3.61 inches.[2] The average length of the vagina (unaroused) is 3 to 5 inches in length. The vagina consists of three layers of tissue—mucous, muscle, and fibrous tissue. During sexual arousal, lubricating fluid discharges through the mucosa. The muscular and fibrous tissue are concentrated around the vaginal opening aids in vaginal contraction and expansion.[3] So, I couldn't imagine a penis being that large going inside anybody's vagina.

Despite all we were experiencing, it felt good to laugh. Knowing that we still possessed the ability to act silly and laugh out-loud about things that seemed to lighten the load during our times of sharing.

To achieve an adequate erection, there must also be properly functioning nerves, arteries, and veins. Disruption to any of these systems can cause erectile dysfunction.[4] Chapter 3 presents the different phases of the human sexual response and its role in sexual function.

CHAPTER 3

Human Sexual Response

Sex on the brain.

The *human sexual response* is the same for women and men. How women and men respond physically and emotionally sexually is not a simple process. In fact, sexual response is not all about his penis all the time. Surprising to most of us including me, a man's brain or thinking plays a more dominate role in sexual function than his penis.[1] Let's examine how each of the three phases of the sexual response are produced and engages the brain and mind.

Sexual Desire and Libido Phase

Sexual desire and libido is having an interest in engaging in sexual activity. Libido is a term used to describe sexual interest and motivation to seek sexual encounters. So, it takes more than just thinking about sex, or fantasizing about it, it's moving beyond the thinking about sex to seeking out an opportunity to engage in sexual activity. In other words, sexual desire and libido are exclusively brain activities without cooperation from the penis at this point. Libido, on the other hand, needs the male hormone testosterone to interact with other brain chemicals such as serotonin, dopamine, and other brain chemicals that work together to control overall mental and physical functioning. Now, I would like to say something that might be a bit confusing. *Testosterone* is not required for an erection to occur, but it sure does help. While testosterone plays a minor role in achieving or maintaining an erection, it remains important for the health and strength of blood vessels and nerves, helping erectile tissue to be suppler. Testosterone also plays a role in the function of the nitric oxide pathway. Under the influence of testosterone more so than without it, the blood vessels are in a much better condition to release nitric oxide, the chemical that stimulates the corpus cavernous smooth muscle as shown in **Figure 2** (page 11), thus resulting in penile erection by smooth muscle relaxation and increased blood flow to the penis. Sexual desire can ebb and flow depending on a number of factors such as age, sex, health, relationship, and life events.[1]

The Sexual Arousal and Erection Phase

Having a desire for sex can set the mood, but arousal jump starts the sexual act, which usually results in erection. Here's where the brain signals the penis to go straight ahead. Arousal is an awareness of sexual stimulation that is usually accompanied by a set of physical responses in which the heart rate increases, breathing quickens, and muscles tense. The body also increases blood flow to nipples and genitals, causing them to harden and swell, and the urethral glands secrete a lubricating fluid. During sexual arousal increased blood flow referred to as vasocongestion causes swelling in the genitals creating an erection. Two erectile bodies in the penis referred to as the corpora cavernosum are actually tubes of tissue that absorbs blood similar to the way a sponge absorbs water. During the excitement phase as the erectile tissue fills with blood, the penis becomes stiff and expands like a balloon filled with water. Impulses from the brain to nerves to veins cause blood to keep the penis erect. Anything that blocks these impulses or restricts blood flow to the penis can cause erectile dysfunction. If blood flow is not restricted, a normal erection is achievable.

During the arousal or excitement phase, there are usually noticeable physical and emotional changes. Muscles continue to tense and vasocongestion reach a peak and the penis releases a few drops of pre-ejaculatory fluid. The arousal phase can last for a few minutes or several hours. The stimuli for arousal can be a response to sight, smell, taste, or sound, a touch, such as an image, a real-life scene, a voice, or fragrance or caress. All stimuli of this nature is considered *psychogenic stimuli*, sources of the first erection because they originate in the brain.

A second type of erection is *reflexogenic* and occurs due to direct genital tactile stimulation. This type of stimulation triggers messengers in the nervous system to travel up the spinal cord and back down again causing an erection. Once again the brain is not critical for controlling these erections, even though a physical response may occur.

The third type of erection is the kind of erection that occurs during sleep referred to as a *nocturnal erection* that also originates in the brain. It's a bit too complicated for me to grasp fully, but here is what I learned. During the sleep cycle, neurochemicals that suppress erections in an awake state release the braking mechanism in the brain to suppress erections. Sexual arousal or excitement on the other hand is characteristic of how excited or turned on one gets when anticipates sex or engaging in it. Arousal is euphoric. In other words, it feels good. Physical sensations associated with arousal include warmth or heat, tingling, blood rushing, and heart pounding.

Sexual desire can ebb and flow depending on a number of factors such as age, sex, health, relationship, and life events. An individual can desire sex, but does not elicit a response that indicates that she/he is turned on. Conversely, men with erectile problems may have no difficulty getting their body to respond physically, but may feel little or no emotional arousal. For example, a male may wake up in the morning with an erection, but not feel sexually turned on. It's also possible to be very sexually aroused and not have an erection. So for men, an erection does not necessarily mean that you are sexually excited or aroused. If the desire for sex and excitement about engaging in sexual activity are present, it is highly likely that an organism is possible.[1]

Orgasm and Ejaculation Phase

Orgasm is the perception of pleasurable sensations with sexual climax. The mind envisioning an image, or anticipating a pleasurable experience is the result of the brain processing a stimuli involving nerves in the pelvic area, which send messages of the increased pressure in the urethra and contractions of the pelvic floor muscles at the base of the penis.

Ejaculation is the physical response to the message, which involves an ejaculatory reflex, nerve signals from the genital and pelvic organs that ascend to the brain and spinal cord and back down. During sex, the ejaculatory ducts contract and force seminal fluid into the urethra and simultaneously close the connection to the bladder neck. During the orgasmic phase, the penis swells and muscles contract involuntarily and rapidly producing an ejaculation. Rapid muscle contractions can also occur in other parts of the body such as the abdomen, thighs, buttocks, feet, and hands. Some spasms may cause the body to tremble. A rash, or "sex flush," may appear over the entire body. Muscles tension subside, as genital organs return to their pre-arousal (flaccid) state. Afterwards, a satisfactory sexual feeling of euphoria occurs due to the pulsations that registering the brain to release oxytocin, which is responsible for the pleasurable feeling of being in love or connected to another person, with or without having sex.

We previously talked about the role of testosterone in penile function and the brain. In the orgasm and ejaculation phase, testosterone's role is that it affects the production of seminal fluid. Men with low levels of testosterone may notice a decrease or less in the amount of fluid released during orgasm. It should be noted that some men who have had their prostate removed can still achieve orgasm without releasing seminal fluid or ejaculate.[1] The next chapter discusses some of the symptoms and causes of erectile dysfunction that can affect penile function.

CHAPTER 4

Symptoms, Causes, and Risk Factors of Erectile Dysfunction

A common reaction: fear of cancer.

Bruce was experiencing prolonged erections more frequently. We didn't know why. Something was causing the blood to remain in his penis for as long as 3-4 hours. When his erections occurred more frequently, without stimulation, I noticed that he began wearing baggy pants and a double layer of long over-sized shirts to cover his pelvic area in case he experienced an erection unexpectedly while teaching or counseling students. After so many episodes, we both knew that a visit to the doctor was long over-due, probably because he feared he was going to be diagnosed with cancer. He didn't want to hear that his erectile problem was the result of the "BIG C", and quite honestly, neither did I.

Despite his fear, Bruce agreed to make an appointment with a urologist located in the Philadelphia area. His 2:00 pm appointment was a week away, which provided plenty of time for me to go online to gather information about symptoms, causes, and risk factors related to erectile dysfunction. Bruce and I visited the urologist in Philadelphia, we had time to review and discuss the following information about symptoms, causes, and risk factors related to erectile dysfunction.

Some Symptoms, Causes, and Risk Factors of Erectile Dysfunction

With ED the most common symptoms include difficulty getting an erection, difficulty keeping an erection, and reduced sexual desire. Experiencing these symptoms from time to time is not cause for alarm. However, if achieving or maintaining an erection happens routinely, it's time to seek medical attention to find a solution to the problem.

When Blood Flow Is Interrupted: Causes and Risk Factors

Both of us knew that an erection occurs when blood fills the penis, but what we didn't know that when blood flow is interrupted, erectile dysfunction often is caused by a combination of factors, not just one as we originally thought. The following is a brief description of some of the factors that may contribute to erectile dysfunction: psychological, neurological, hormonal, arterial, and venous.

Psychological Causes of Erectile Dysfunction

Psychological factors that may lead to ED include depression, performance anxiety, stress, mental disorders, stress, and relationship problems. Most times medications are prescribed to address psychological issues, which can also contribute to erection problems.[1]

Neurological Causes of Erectile Dysfunction

Nerves play an important role in carrying messages to all parts of the body including the pelvic area. Operations in the pelvic area including the prostate cancer, bladder, colon, and radiation may result in nerve damage and debilitating loss of sexual function. Operations to the pelvic area can also increase a man's risk for ED. In addition neurological (nerve and brain) diseases such as stroke, multiple sclerosis (MS), Alzheimer's disease, Parkinson's disease, and spinal cord injuries are common for men who experience erectile dysfunction. These diseases may interrupt the transmission of nerve impulses between the brain and penis.[2]

Hormonal Causes of Erectile Dysfunction

As men age, hormone levels decrease naturally. When testosterone levels decrease, a broad range of symptoms occur including a decrease in energy and sexual interest which drives most men to seek testing. There are several hormonal tests that measure key hormones known to play an important role in men's overall health, including tests for testosterone and prolactin levels. *Testosterone* is the primary sex hormone and anabolic steroid in males. Testosterone plays a key role in the development of male reproductive tissues such as testes and prostate, as well as promoting secondary sexual characteristics such as increased muscle and bone mass, and the growth of body hair. Low testosterone can contribute to ED but rarely is the sole factor responsible for ED.

Another hormonal test includes a *Sex Hormone Binding Globulin Test* (SHBG), which is used to find out how much testosterone, estrogen, and dihydotestosterone is going in body tissue. This particular test requires a blood test through needle injection. Some factors that can affect low levels of testosterone include obesity, type 2 diabetes, HIV, age, and medications.

An additional measure to determine the level of testosterone is the *Prolactin Test*, which helps to find the cause of a man's low sex drive/or erectile dysfunction. Test results can provide information on the hormone level and whether levels are normal, low, or high.[3]

Medications

Certain prescription drugs and over-the-counter drugs can cause ED. Drugs that can cause possible side effects that may influence sexual function include diuretics, pills that increase urine flow, high blood pressure meds, antidepressants, tranquilizers, muscle relaxers, prostate cancer drugs, and hormones are some of the drugs that can influence sexual function. When visiting your urologist, it is very important to inform the doctor about all the drugs you take, including nonprescription drugs. All of these substances can damage blood vessels and/or restrict blood flow to the penis, causing ED.[4]

Veinous and Arterial Causes of Erectile Dysfunction

Sexual function in men and women incorporates physiologic processes and regulation of the central and peripheral nervous systems, the vascular system, and the endocrine system. In order to achieve an erection the nerves to the penis must be functioning properly, the blood circulation to the penis must be functioning properly, and there must be a stimulus from the brain. If something interferes with any of these conditions, a full erection can be difficult to achieve or maintain. If the veins in the penis cannot prevent blood from leaving the penis during an erection, an erection cannot be maintained. This is known as a *venous leak*, and can be a result of injury, disease, or stress. Some common vascular diseases that affect blood vessels include atherosclerosis (hardening of the arteries) can affect the artery and vein that supplies blood to the penis which is much narrower than the artery to the heart. Conditions that affect cardiovascular health can also affect sexual function.[5]

High Blood Pressure

Hypertension (high blood pressure and high cholesterol), another vascular disease can restrict blood flow to the heart, the brain, and the penis. If the veins in the penis cannot prevent blood from leaving the penis during an erection, an erection cannot be maintained. This is known as a *venous leak*, and can be a result of injury, disease, or stress.[6]

Diabetes

Diabetes can also cause nerve damage and artery damage that can make achieving an erection difficult. High glucose levels or diabetes can damage the small blood vessels in the body, including those supplying blood to the pelvic area.[7]

Kidney Disease

Kidney disease can cause chemical changes that affect hormones, circulation, nerve function, and energy level. These changes have the potential to lower libido (sex drive) or sexual ability. Taking drugs to manage kidney disease may be a risk factor for erectile dysfunction.[8]

Other Possible Causes of Erectile Dysfunction

Erectile dysfunction can be caused by life-style issues related to poor diet, excessive use of tobacco, smoking, and obesity, and even cycling. *Cycling* is a popular mode of exercise for men and women. However, men who bike can experience erectile problems as a consequence of spending too much time on a bike seat. Researchers have discovered that some male cyclists develop damage to the *pudendal nerve*, the main nerve in the perineum, and the pudendal artery which sends blood to the penis. Men who spend a lot of hours on a bike have reported numbness and trouble achieving an erection. Over time, erectile problems occur when arteries and nerves get caught between the narrow bicycle seat and the rider's pubic bones. Injury or trauma to the penis as well as chronic illness, certain medications, a condition called *Peyronie's disease* (scar tissue in the penis) may be contributing factors. Modifying life-style issues can be effective in reducing or eliminating the risk of ED.[9]

Knowing When to Seek Help

Knowing when to seek help is important. While most men are reluctant to talk about erectile concerns for fear of a cancer diagnosis. Not all erectile dysfunction issues are the result of a cancerous condition. Speaking to the doctor can help you and your partner determine if your partner's erectile dysfunction is psychological, or medically related. It's more than likely that the cause of erectile dysfunction is far more complex than what you imagined. No matter how complex the situation, there is hope. Your urologist can help you and your partner decide on which available treatment options are most effective in managing your particular problem. Chapter 5 includes a discussion of current and innovative treatment options.

CHAPTER 5

Current Treatment Options

*Finding a solution for ED may feel like
trying to find a needle in a haystack.*

E rectile dysfunction (ED) is a common condition affects over 3 million men in the United States every year. Given the prevalence of severe co-morbidities associated with ED, the clinician must take a through history and conduct a diagnostic exam accordingly. The clinician should consider that every man who presents with ED is unique in regards to symptoms, degree of stress, associated health conditions, sexual relationship, quality, and sociocultural context. The clinician determines an appropriate treatment plan that is aligned with the patient's and his partner's priorities and values, adopting a shared decision-making process.

The American Urology Association guideline acknowledges noninvasive and invasive treatment options including oral phoshodiesterase type 5 inhibitors (PDE5i), vacuum erection devices (VED), intracavernosa injections (ICI), intraurethral suppositories, and penile prosthesis for ED.

Novel approaches to treat ED, including but not limited to extracorporeal shock wave therapy (ESWT), penile vascular surgeries, stem cell therapies (SCT), and platelet-rich-plasma (PRP), have shown promising results and may become more commonly suggested by clinicians.[1]

The following is a review of current medical and surgical treatment options, as well as innovative therapeutic options in ED begins with noninvasive options that are usually suggested by clinicians as first-line therapy for patients.

Non Invasive First Line Treatment Options

Life-Style Modifications

Some modifications in life-style can have a positive impact on erection function. Effective life-style modifications may include weight loss, proper diet and daily exercise, weight control, stress management, or relationship counseling. Your doctor may recommend sex therapy. Sex therapy is a form of relationship counseling that may help a man if his physical exams and blood tests are normal. Sex therapy may also be effective in dealing with financial worries, relationship conflicts, and communication issues. The therapist may give you and your partner some homework, such as touching exercises designed to take away the pressure to perform during sex, or ways to improve communication skills before, during, and after sexual intimacy. Your doctor will help you and your partner explore the possibility of life-style modification as an effective treatment for improving erectile function.

Oral PDE5i Medications

In addition to life-style modifications, oral phosphodiesterase type 5 inhibitors (PDE5i) including Viagra (sidenafil), Cialis (tadalafil), Avanafil (stendra), and Vardenafil (staxyn) have been preferred as front-line therapies for patients. Up to 65% of men who are taking PDE5i show a successful rate of sexual intercourse after initial treatment.[2,3] However, it should be noted that underlying effects of ED related to radiation and co-morbidities such as diabetes can decrease the success rate of PDE5i.[4-7] Additional testing and specialist referral are options reserved for cases where initial treatments failed. Younger patients with a history of pelvic trauma, significant penile deformity, complicated diseases affecting endocrine glands, complicated psychiatric or psychosexual disorders, need for vascular or neurological intervention, and medicolegal reasons are examples of other indications for specialist referral.[8]

Nitric oxide (NO) plays a role in the physiology of the penis, operating chiefly as the principal mediator of erectile function. The presence of NO stimulates the corpus cavernous smooth muscle as shown in **Figure 2** (page 11), resulting in penile erection by smooth muscle relaxation and increased blood flow to the penis. Alterations in the biology of NO likely account for variations in erectile dysfunction. In regard to PDE5i, without the induction of penile erection via NO release PDE5i are not effective. Nor do PDE5i work sufficiently in diabetic neuropathy or cavernous nerve damage from pelvic surgeries, such as radical prostatectomy or other pelvic surgeries, due to lack of NO release.[9]

Regarding PDE5i as first line therapy, the starting lowest dose should be prescribed, and closely monitored for effectiveness as well as side effects. All have different biological and pharmacological properties, but similar effectiveness. Viagra (sidenanafil), and Vardenafil (staxyn) duration of action is 10-12 hours, and is absorbed within 30-60 minutes. Eating fatty foods will reduce their effectiveness, and should be taken 1 hour before eating and 2 hours after eating to receive maximum absorption. Stendra (avanafil) is absorbed 15-30 minutes with a duration of action up to 6 hours. Cialis (tadalafil's) action of duration is 24-36 hours with a longer onset of action 60-120 minutes. A bit of good news is avanafil and tadalafil are not affected by food intake, and tadalafil is the only oral medication approved by the U.S. Food and Drug Administration to be used daily to treat ED, as well as lower urinary tract symptoms and benign prostatic hyperplasia.[9]

If total testosterone levels are low, PDESi treatment for ED may require combination therapy with testosterone to improve effectiveness.[10, 11]

Vacuum erection device (VED)

The *VED* is a mechanical device that is placed over the penis to generate negative pressure to pull blood into the penis and cause an erection. A rubberized band is placed around the base of the penis to maintain the erection during sexual intercourse, **Figure 3** (page 29). It is effective for men with ED associated with diabetes, spinal cord injury, post-prostatectomy, and other conditions. The satisfaction rate was reported up to 90%. However, the discontinuation rate was up to

30% due to pain and temporary changes in to penile sensations due to the rubberized band and ejaculation problems. Bruising can also occur if the device is over pressurized, bruising, pain and temporary changes to penile sensation may result. In addition, its use may be difficult for patients with insufficient dexterity or a large amount of lower abdominal fat and buried penis.[12-15]

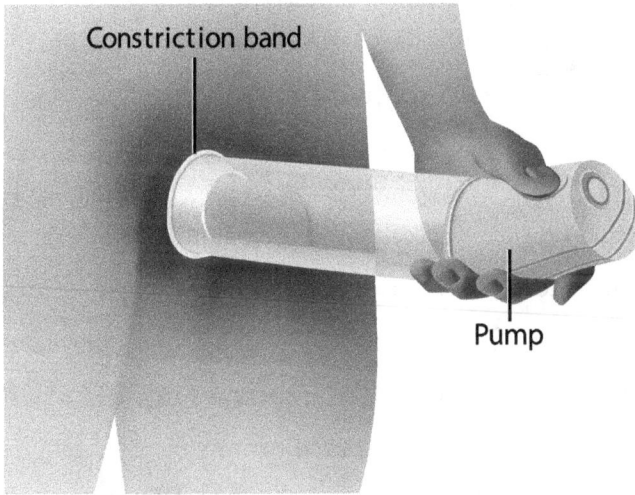

Constriction band

Pump

Figure 3: *Vacuum Erection Device.*

Intraurethral Alprostadil (MUSE): A Self-Inserted Suppository

Alprostadil is a small suppository that comes preloaded in an applicator that's inserted into the urethra. The applicator is placed in the tip of the penis, and the small button on the side of the applicator is pressed releasing the suppository. Gently rubbing the penis dissolves the suppository in the urethra, and the medication is absorbed. The medication increases smooth muscles cells causing blood flow and leading to a penile erection. The most side effect is burning or pain, and men who have undergone radical prostatectomy seem to have an increased incidence of discomfort.[16] A test dose of medication should be administered in the clinic with patient to monitor for hypotension and other adverse side effects such as penile pain and urethral burning.[17] Success rate for sexual intercourse is 39-60%.[18]

This route of administration may be a good option for who do not prefer injection methods or cannot use oral medications due to contributing factors or contraindications.[19]

Intracavernosal (ICI) Self Injection

A medication can directly be injected into the corpus cavernosum from the lateral base of the penis. The most commonly used medication for ICI is alprostadil, which is the only FDA approved medication to be used for ICI, **Figure 4** (page 31). Alprostadil can also be combined with other medications to receive higher efficacy. ICI is an alternative treatment for oral ED therapy with better satisfaction rates up to 94% and minimal systemic side effects.[20-21]

The fear of administering the drug by injection in the penis causes anxiety, which makes the administration a bit more challenging compared to other options. The first dose should be administered in the clinic to determine the optimal dose to achieve a good erection that does not last longer than 1 hour. The man and his partner should be counseled regarding the potential use of ICI therapy which may result in priapism (painful prolonged erections), with bruising. Patients with Peyronie's disease, a history of recurrent priapism and bleeding disorders, may be at risk for ICI.[22]

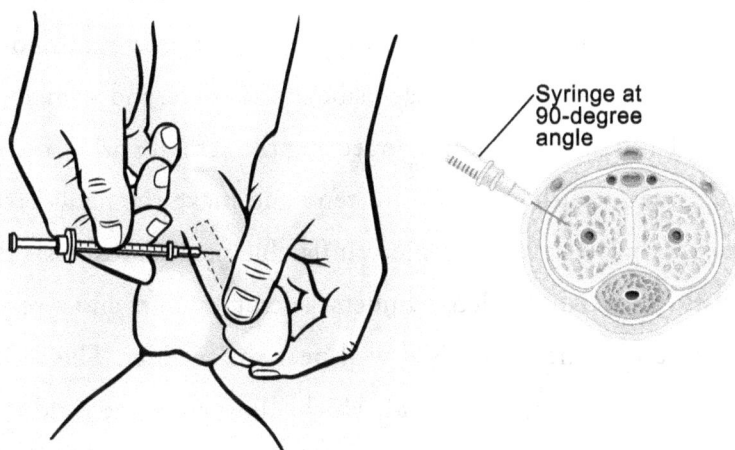

Figure 4: *Intracavernosal Injection internal view of corpora cavernosum*

Invasive Treatment Options Requiring Surgery

Penile Prothesis Implants

The *penile prosthesis* is a surgically implanted device that has been used for ED treatment over the last 40 years. There are multiple forms of penile prosthesis, including the semi-rigid prosthesis device and inflatable devices. In **Figure 5** (page 32), the semi-rigid device contains two-semi-rigid cylinders that are implanted into the penile corpora. The semi-rigid is ideal for patients who are physically handicapped with poor hand dexterity.[23] The semi-rigid prosthesis remains the same width at all times; you bend the penis up when you wish to have intercourse and down to conceal the penis.[24]

There are two types of inflatable penile prosthesis that consist of either two or three pieces. The two-piece prosthesis is composed of two cylinders, one placed in each side of the penis, and a small pump that is placed in the scrotum. Squeezing the scrotal pushes fluid into the cylinders, causing them to distend and make the penis erect. In **Figure 6** (below) the three-piece inflatable penile prosthesis device consists of two fluid-filled cylinders, a scrotal pump, and a reservoir that fits under the abdominal wall near the bladder. The reservoir contains a large amount of fluid, which allows for more rigidity than is possible with the two-piece unit. The patient satisfaction rate of IPP are 86% that is higher than oral medication or ICI [guideline]. The 5 and 10 year overall survivals of modern prosthetics are estimated to bo be 90.4% and 86.6%, respectively.[25]

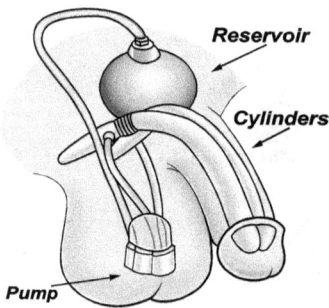

Figure 5: *2-piece Inflatable implant*   **Figure 6:** *3-piece Inflatable implant*

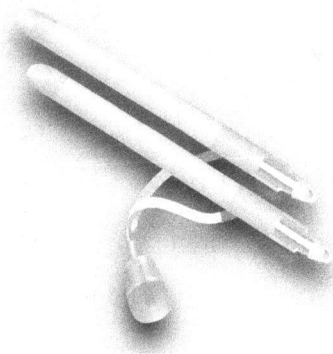

Penile vascular surgery

Penile arterial reconstruction surgery may be considered for young patients who do not have any evidence of generalized vascular disease, or other co-morbidities that could compromise vascular integrity.[26]

There have been numerous controversies due to the absence of large prospective and well-controlled studies. Also, long term success of the procedure is not well established.[27]

Intracavernosal stem cell therapy (SCT)

Mesenchymal stem cells are adult stem cells that have regenerative effects for a variety of medical conditions. Currently, mesenchymal stem cells isolated from adipose tissue are the most frequently used cells in studies. These cells are capable of differentiating into a variety of cells, such as cavernosal smooth muscle cells, endothelial cells, or neuron cells, that can provide cell growth and survival.[28-31] There are several clinical in small study groups that have shown promising results using SCT without significant adverse effects in diabetic and post-prostatectomy ED.[32,33] Further randomized controlled studies are warranted with long-term follow up periods, standardized protocols, and larger study groups.

Extracorporeal shock wave therapy (ESWT)

Low intensity extracorporeal shock wave therapy is a novel modality developed for treating ED. Extracorporeal shock wave therapy is thought to induce cellular microtrauma, which in turn stimulates angiogenic factors that promote blood vessel growth factors, restoration and repair of tissue. ESWT has not been approved by the FDA and is still under investigation. However, several studies had reported its efficacy and safety in mild to moderate vasculogenic ED when PDE5i (oral medications) failed.[34-36] However well-designed prospective randomized clinical trials are limited in the literature. The duration of treatment, efficacy, optimal treatment parameters, such as dosing frequency, energy flux density settings, and the number of shocks, and the selection of device types (linear versus focused shock wave) are not well established. Randomized controlled studies with larger sample sizes are needed to determine its long-term efficacy and side effects using a validated and standard protocol.[37]

Platelet-rich plasma (PRP) and other therapies

Platelet-rich plasma is a blood product that contains a high amount of platelets with various growth factors, including platelet-derived growth factor (PDGF), insulin-like growth, fibroblast (FGF), and vascular endothelial growth factor (VEGF), all of which have been shown to induce cell regeneration, proliferation, and differentiation in preclinical and clinical studies.[38-42] There has been some success in phase I human trials with 17 patients with ED and Peyronie's disease. Results showed no major adverse effect. However, PRP is considered an experimental treatment, and higher-quality randomized controlled studies with larger patient samples with a logn term follow-up are needed.

The majority of patients with ED start off on oral treatments with PDE5i as initial therapy. Before staring PDE5i, the clinician should provide easy to understand instructions to maximize benefits and efficacy. No matter choice of treatment, your urologist should consider your medical history and sociocultural background. Improvements in existing therapies developed over the last decade, such as stem cell therapy (SCT) therapy, gene therapy, and plasma-rich platelet therapy (PRP) may replace or regenerate cells in the penis. However, well-designed randomized controlled studies with standardized protocols and larger study populations are needed.

In addition new pharmacologic agents targeting underlying pathologies that affect penile function are promising therapies based on preclinical studies. The implementation of novel surgical treatments using tissue transplants and new device-base treatments such as novel drug and drug delivery are possible ED therapies in the future.[43]

A word of caution. I advise you and your partner to not become too fixated on anyone solution or treatment option until the urologist does a thorough examination that includes your partner's medical history, sociocultural background, and a discussion about all possible choices including lifestyle modification and mental health counseling for anxiety or communication issues with your partner that may correct the problem. The choice of treatment option is one that is based on shared decision making between doctor, patient, and patient's partner.

CHAPTER 6

The Initial Diagnosis

Duo is better than solo.

We arrived at the clinic before our 2:00 o'clock appointment only to be told it was pushed back until 3:00 o'clock because the doctor had not arrived yet. Anticipating a delay in seeing the doctor, we were glad we remembered taking a few necessary items that came in handy during our visit to the doctor.

How to Prepare for the Doctor's Visit

1. Before the doctor's appointment, do your homework. Go on the Internet to view the doctor's publications including books and articles and memberships in organizations. If available, listen to a YouTube presentation, take note of any patient reviews and ratings including photos of your doctor. Then share information with your partner, all of which will help you and your partner to become better acquainted with the doctor before your appointment.

2. Bring a pocket notebook. The night before the visit or on the way to the doctor's office, talk to your partner about the symptoms he is experiencing, and record them in a pocket notebook. Record

symptoms that he thinks are related and not related like decreased appetite, insomnia, frequent trips to the bathroom.

3. Prior to visiting the doctor, take note of all the medications including vitamins, herbal remedies and take them with you when you visit the doctor. Make sure you record them in the notebook along with the dosage, and time of day administered.

4. Take pocket change for coffee or snacks in case you leave home early and have to skip breakfast or stay later than expected.

5. Take your favorite magazine to read to pass the time while you wait for the doctor's arrival.

When we entered the doctor's office, we noticed his bedside manner. It was pleasant. He greeted us, shook our hands, and invited us to make ourselves comfortable before asking Bruce a series of questions: *How long have you had the erection, How often do they occur, How long do they normally last, Have you used drugs, legal or illegal, Did the symptoms occur after an injury, Do you have sickle cell or anyone in your immediate family?* Bruce said he was not a drug user nor did he have sickle cell or a known history of sickle cell in his family. After answering all the questions, he prepared to take the physical exam and whatever blood tests were necessary. I voluntarily left the room.

The physical included an examination of the genitals, a *digital rectal examination*, a series of blood tests, including a prostate specific antigen test to determine the health of the prostate and a *Gleason Test* to predict how fast prostate cancer is growing, the doctor reported what he suspected: priapism.

The First Diagnosis: When It's Priapism

What is *Priapism*? Priapism is a persistent erection that continues hours beyond sexual stimulation, or without sexual stimulation. Priapism develops when blood is trapped in the penis and is unable to drain. The doctor said that priapism was relatively rare. In most cases, priapism occurs in men who suffer from blood disorders, especially *sickle cell* disease. Unlike healthy blood cells that are smooth, round, bendable and can easily flow through blood vessels and carry oxygen to every part of the body, sickled cells are irregular-shaped and do not carry oxygen well, which can result in diminished oxygen delivery to organs causing sexual dysfunction and other complications **Figure 7** (below).

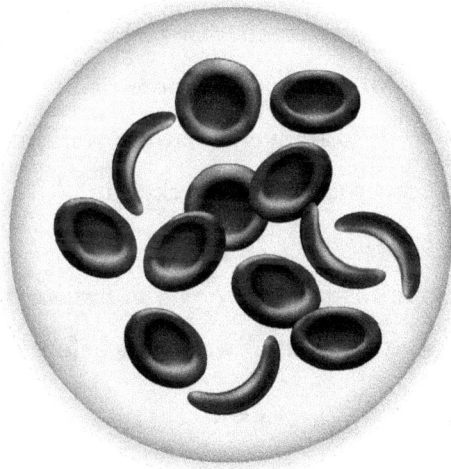

Figure 7: *Healthy red blood cells and sickle cells*

Even some medications can put some men at higher risk. In rare cases, priapism can affect children with sickle cell. If left untreated, scarring and permanent erectile dysfunction could occur.[1]

As we prepared to leave the doctor's office, Bruce was told to continue to monitor the erections, and go immediately to the emergency room for treatment.

The prolonged erections continued for many weeks after the initial doctor's visit. The erections lasted sometime more than four hours at a time. Never knowing when an erection might occur, he never slept soundly. He was worried about having an erection that would require another trip to the emergency room. Sometimes he wouldn't drift off until early morning, which meant he was going to work worried about when he would have to go back to the emergency room.

When It Won't Go Down

It seemed as if Bruce was experiencing an erection sometimes twice a day. The erections were becoming more painful. The visits to the emergency room were so frequent that the staff on duty knew why we were there before Bruce was checked in. After going through registration, he was assigned a room and told that the doctor would be in shortly to administer *aspiration and irrigation* of the penis, a procedure we knew little about. It was hours before assistance arrived.

By the time the doctor and his medical team arrived, Bruce was grimacing with pain. I moved to the side of the room to make ample space for the healthcare professionals to surround the hospital bed and busy themselves setting up equipment. While the healthcare professionals were preparing for the procedure, I was preparing to ask questions about the procedure and record the responses in a small pocket notebook that I brought with me.

The doctor introduced himself and then proceeded to ask the same stream of questions as the last doctor: how long do the erections usually last, any known trauma to the pelvic area, any excessive use of recreational drugs including alcohol, have you been here before, do you have a urologist, are you on any medications. Bruce answered all of questions, after which the doctor began to explain the procedure, and use of equipment required during the procedure.

Equipment for the procedure included sterile gloves, an antimicrobial solution used to sterilize the entire penile area, anesthesia to numb the penis, several syringes and needles for saline flushes and phenylephrine injections used to facilitate draining of the corpora cavernosa, a towel to drape near the base of the penis to absorb any excess drainage of blood from the penis, and gauze and self-adherent tape to be applied over the puncture at the base of the penis when the procedure is completed.

I watched the medical professionals under the leadership of the doctor move as rhythmic as a musical group lead by a conductor. After several attempts to drain the penis using the solutions provided, nothing much happened. Bruce's penis was still enlarged. The small amount of blood that drained from his penis was not nearly enough to provide the relief needed. After repeated failed attempts, the doctor started to gently squeeze the penis intermittently several times to increase blood flow from the penis. The blood appeared very thick and dark like grape jelly, and seemed to come out in clumps. Using a small sterilized kidney-shaped basin to deposit excess blood, the doctor continued to exert pressure on the penis. After several laborious hours, Bruce's penis returned to its normal size, and gauze and self-adhesive tape was placed over the injection site to prevent blood leakage.

Feeling emotionally and physically drained, Bruce laid there for a while until we were told we could leave, at which time the doctor returned and instructed him to return if the erection returns.

A few days later, the erections returned. Bruce went through the same procedure again. After his last episode, he made what was to be his final appointment with his local urologist who told him that aspiration and irrigation was not an effective treatment for him. He recommended two recourses. One recourse was surgery to insert an *inflatable prosthesis*, which was not a welcomed solution. Bruce's response, "No way. I'm not going out like that." I just sat there silently waiting on the doctor to offer the other solution because the one offered was a no go. To our dismay, no other treatment options were provided. After seeing our disappointment, the doctor then offered another option. He said,

> There's a nationally and internationally known expert in the field of urology, Dr. Arthur Burnett. He's located at Johns Hopkins Medical Center in Baltimore, Maryland. He's an expert in the field of urology. He may be able to help you because there are other treatments for priapism.

We thanked the doctor, and gladly took his advice. We scheduled an appointment immediately after we returned home. The drive back to Philadelphia gave us plenty of time to think about planning ahead.

CHAPTER 7

The Second Diagnosis

Know who you're dealing with.

As soon as we returned home, we wasted no time preparing for the five hour trip to Baltimore. Planning ahead of the appointment also provided time for me to once again go on the Internet to review Dr. Burnett's credentials. In addition, his most recent book, *The Manhood Every Man's Guide to Improving Sexual Heath and Overall Wellness* included his early career aspirations as a urologist and his astounding list of accomplishment.[1]

During his post-graduate training in early 1990s, Dr. Burnett's research examined how nitric oxide, a gaseous molecule generated inside the body can act as a neurotransmitter—a nervous system chemical messenger—when it is released from the nerve supplying the penis to control erections. Previous neuroscience over decades had failed to identify the actual neurotransmitter in nerves that converge in the penis for mediating penile stimulation. Dr. Burnett's research led him to the project that helped clarify how nitric oxide works to further drive penile erection. The science of nitric oxide biology in the penis has since been recognized as a major advance in medicine.

A direct result of this progress was the development of Vigra and Cialis for the treatment of ED.

Dr. Burnett is a Distinguished Professor of Urology with the Johns Hopkins University School of Medicine, home to the oldest and most distinguished urology department in the country. With over 30 years of experience as an urologist, he is considered an internationally acclaimed urologist and one of the prominent authorities in the field. He is director of the Male Consultation Clinic at Johns Hopkins Hospital, a clinician-scientist at the James Buchanan Brady Urological Institute. He also directs the Basic Science Laboratory in Neurology at the Johns Hopkins School of Medicine. He is an expert in the areas of prostate cancer, urinary tract malignancies, urinary tract reconstruction, erectile dysfunction, and penile abnormalities, and female urology as well as having performed over 2,000 radical prostatectomies.

He was the lead urologic surgeon on the John Hopkins team that performed the first-ever penis/pelvic transplant. He has written more than 500 original peer-review articles, scientific reviews, editorials, and book chapters, appearing in prominent journals such as *Science, Nature, Medicine, Proceedings of the National Academy of Sciences, Journal of Urology, Urology,* and *Journal of Andrology.* He has received countless honors for his stellar work in the urology field, and he is a member of over 30 notable organizations in the field, such as The American Urological Association, American Medical Association, and International Society for the study of Women's Sexual Health, to name a few. As a world-authority in the science and medicine of erectile dysfunction, Dr. Burnett has also paved the way for the clinical development of oral medications to treat erectile dysfunction such as Viagra as mentioned earlier. After reviewing his credentials, we both gave Dr. Burnett our seal of approval. We were excited about meeting him in person and hoped that his bedside manner was as impressive as his accomplishments.

When It's Time For a Second Opinion

By the time we arrived in Baltimore, our early rising at 4:00am coupled with the 5-hour drive to Baltimore left us both a bit weary. The greeting we received revived us. We were pleasantly surprised to be greeted by a middle age African American male who served as the receptionist. His friendly manner of welcoming us was very noticeable. His pleasant smile, sturdy handshake, and the casual conversation were delightfully professional but genuine. While we made ourselves comfortable, we couldn't help but notice the large group of diverse men waiting to be seen by the doctor. Most of whom appeared to be older African American men around Bruce's age. Bruce was surprised to see so many men seeking help who looked like him. A little later the receptionist announced to everyone in the waiting room that the doctor was running behind, and he would be in within the next hour. Within the hour the doctor did return, and we were called back.

When we saw Dr. Burnett, we exhaled silently. Even though we saw Dr. Burnett's picture on the Internet and knew before coming that he was a man of color, somehow we were still surprised. The doctor, like most of his clients, appeared to be African American. The feeling we both had was the kind of feeling one gets when you have read great things about someone you admire, and you finally get the chance to meet them in person. I was beaming inside with pride, and knowing Bruce, I knew he was too. Dr. Burnett greeted us, shook our hands, and asked about our trip to Baltimore. He then expressed how pleased he was to see partners attend the initial doctor's visit. We introduced ourselves, and casually chatted about our plans to retire soon. I noticed that he didn't rush the conversation or give the impression that we were on a time clock, even though the waiting room was thriving with clients waiting to see him.

After introductions the doctor prepared to conduct a physical exam that included an examination of the genitals, *biopsy*, and blood tests that indicated his *PSA levels* were elevated and showed signs of cancerous cells. Bruce was diagnosed with late prostate cancer[2,3] which was a shock to the both of us. Bruce didn't know he had cancer nor did I.

As a health educator, I know that the prostate-specific antigen is a protein produced by normal prostate cells. PSA also produces cancerous and non-cancerous tissue in the prostate, a small gland that sits below the bladder. The highest amount of PSA is found in the seminal fluid; some PSA is also found in the serum, the fluid component of blood that includes all proteins, electrolytes, antibodies, and antigens not used in blood clotting.[4-6] Rising levels of serum are associated with prostate cancer.[7] I also know that the prostate-specific antigen test is used primarily to screen for prostate cancer by measuring the level of prostate-specific antigen in the blood.

But what I didn't know was that according to Dr. Burnett, Bruce's former doctor prescribed a testosterone blocker, an anti-androgen to shut down the ability to have an erection, which probably was a viable solution to priapism at the time. However, long-term use of the hormone prohibited the prostate tissue from producing prostate-specific antigen, which in turn deflated or masked his PSA level so that the presence of cancer went undetected resulting in the timely diagnosis and treatment for prostate cancer.[8]

According to Dr. Burnett, anti-androgen therapies have been used, often with fairly good success, as they are thought to block androgen-dependent, sleep related erections that precede priapism episode. However, anti-androgen therapies are associated with multiple long-term side effects including mood changes, decreased libido, physical growth abnormalities, adverse cardiovascular effects, and impaired reproductive function. For these reasons, before administering anti-androgen therapies, clinicians should counsel patients on potential risks and benefits.[9, 10]

As a result of Bruce's unexpected cancer diagnosis, surgery was recommended as soon as possible. The surgical plan was to remove as much of the cancerous tissue around the prostate without removing the prostate.

When You Have Questions

The *prostate cancer diagnosis* was the beginning of a real plan of action with a healthcare team. To feel more organized I brought a notebook to record all important information including the responses to our many questions as well as upcoming appointments, and test results. The old adage, "two is company and three is a crowd," does not apply when seeking help for an erectile condition that affects you and your partner. Having more information together helped to relieve some of the stress of the prostate cancer diagnosis. Here is helpful information that I obtained from the ZERO-the End of Prostate Cancer website, www.zerpcancer.org/learn.

Questions For Your Doctor
Diagnosis

1. What exactly is my diagnosis?

2. What is the stage, PSA level and Gleason score?

3. How aggressive is the cancer?

4. What other tests will be done?

Treatment

1. What are all my treatment options?

2. What is the goal of treatment?

3. What treatment do you recommend based on my stage?

4. Why do you recommend this particular treatment?

5. Am I eligible for a clinical trial?

6. What are the potential side effects of the treatment we discussed?

7. How can these side effects be managed?

8. What will my treatment schedule be?

Living with Prostate Cancer

1. Are my siblings, children, and grandchildren at higher risk?

2. What steps can I take to be active and healthy during and after treatment?

3. Are there resources or services for my spouse or partner?

4. How will treatment affect my sexual function?

> *Note: This information is published by ZERO-the End of Prostate cancer. Use it in your conversations with your health care team about prostate cancer and related topics. For more information about prostate cancer and ZERO-the End of Prostate Cancer, visit www.zerpcancer.org/learn. This information is a service provided by ZERO-the End of Prostate Cancer. It is not intended to take the place of medical professionals or the recommendation of your healthcare team. ZERO- the End of Prostate Cancer strongly suggest consulting your healthcare team if you have questions about specific care.*

After the consultation, we scheduled the appointment for surgery to take place in two weeks. During the drive back to Philadelphia, neither one of us said a word. On the drive back to Philadelphia we were silent. It wasn't until we were home that we discussed the diagnosis, looked over the information recorded in my notebook, and revisited our confidence in Dr. Burnett, that we agreed that all would be well.

We spent the next few days preparing for the return trip to the hospital. We sat down together every evening to review the list of items we wanted to take with us. You and your partner should probably do the same as we discovered two heads are better than one, especially when trying to remember all the important items we probably would have forgotten if we had not prepared ahead of time.

When planning to stay in the hospital, it is important to be prepared. Making a list of items ahead of time will help you and your partner think through what you need to take with you so you're not stuck doing without needed items. I also want to remind you that most hospitals will not take responsibility if personal items are stolen. You may want to call ahead of time to find out if the hospital offers lockable storage in the rooms.

How To Prepare For an Overnight Stay at the Hospital

1. **Clothing:** pajamas, slippers, socks, undergarments, an outfit to wear home

2. **Personal care products:** eyeglasses, medications, soap, hair care products, toothpaste, tooth brush, and deodorant, earplugs

3. **Electronic equipment:** Laptop, cell phone and charger, favorite book or magazine

4. **Sundry items:** Book of inspirational readings for meditation while waiting for surgery results, favorite book or magazine plus a pocket notebook to record medical prescriptions and aftercare required after surgery, and future appointments

5. **Small food and drink items:** Bottled water, favorite pre-packaged snacks. These items also come in handy when traveling.

6. **Room reservation:** If you made reservations at a nearby hotel, confirm reservations before you depart. I had planned on staying at a nearby hotel while in Baltimore, but decided to stay overnight

in the hospital room with Bruce. Be prepared to be uncomfortable as the only sleeping accommodation was a narrow declining chair that folded down. You may want to ask a head of time if the hospital provides sleeping accommodations for partners.

CHAPTER 8
Day of Surgery

All things work together for good...

Although we drove to Baltimore the day before surgery, we decided not to drive to the hospital the day of surgery despite the short walking distance from the hotel to the hospital. Since Bruce was starting to experience intermittent pain in his legs making it difficult for him to walk or stand at times, I decided it would be a good idea to reserve the hotel shuttle vehicle to take us to the hospital the day of surgery to avoid traffic and the hassle of finding a parking space.

That evening I walked to a nearby restaurant and ordered two seafood dinners while Bruce stayed behind to rest. When I returned, we sat on the edge of the bed to eat our meals then retired early to rise long before daybreak.

Early in the morning Bruce got up to go to the bathroom as usual. His stirring was an indication for me to get up with him in case he needed assistance. When he tried to stand, he immediately fell back on the bed. He sat there for a moment and tried to gather himself to stand on his own, but he could not. He looked at me, and I could see tears of hopelessness well in his eyes. We had no idea what was happening. I knew we needed help. I immediately called the main desk to request a wheel chair, and provided instructions for the van to be ready to transport us to the hospital shortly. When the wheel chair arrived, Bruce tried to lift himself once again without my assistance, but he couldn't. Frustrated, he sat down heavily on the bed, "I can't do this," he said. "Yes, you can," I replied. Determined, I convinced him that on the count of three, we were going to use our combined strength to lift him into the chair. We did.

At daybreak the air was exceedingly cold, and the sky gray. No sun or hint of sun. It was 6:00 a.m. when we arrived at the hospital. Bruce signed in after which an attendant arrived to take Bruce to his hospital room in preparation for surgery. As he was slowly wheeled away, we glanced at each other and gave a reassuring smile indicating everything would be ok. I waited until the attendant called me back to Bruce. Since we arrived early, there was plenty of time for us to talk before surgery.

While we waited, to my surprise my son Patrick arrived. I had called him before we left Philadelphia to inform him about Bruce's surgery. When he arrived, he extended his hand to Bruce in support by offering prayer. As we joined hands, Bruce was surprised by the gesture and was brought to tears as we prayed. I was grateful Patrick came. Soon afterwards, an attendant arrived to take Bruce to surgery, and I took the elevator to the waiting room.

When I entered the waiting area, there seemed a dark covering of gray over the waiting room, a quiet and subtle gloom that made the room and other family members waiting there appear dark, probably due to the absence of sunlight.

When the doctor arrived, he asked me how I was doing. "Fine. I'm just a tad tired from not sleeping well last night," I said. He nodded his head indicating that he understood. I paused, and he started talking softly about how long the procedure and recovery time would take. Afterwards, he asked me if I had any questions. "Just one," I said. "Doctor, are you a praying man?" I asked. He was a little surprised but because the question was asked in a flash, he did not hesitate to do the same. He immediately replied,

> A few days before surgery and the day of surgery, I read over the patient's file. I make sure I go to bed early so I'm well rested the day of surgery. In the am before the operation, I pray for God's guidance, and then I meet with the family to let them know how long the surgery will take bar any unexpected complications.

His response was reassuring. Once again I had no doubt that we had the best doctor for the job.

When Meditation Helps

After the doctor left, I settled back in the waiting room. I noticed the quiet hum of family members whispering to one other as they waited to hear from their loved one's doctor and the distant ding of elevators going up and down seemed to lull me to sleep. Somehow it was comforting to know that life was still going on around me. An hour had passed and quiet hums were making me anxious. While I waited, I could do one of two things. I could stay where I was and worry. That was unproductive or I could reminisce about the *joys of life* including the time when Bruce and I first met, and the many ways God has been good to me down through the years. That was peaceful.

We met in a group home where worked as a clinical counselor for at-risk teens, and I was a houseparent, a staff member who supervised children in a court-ordered residential placement. I remembered how painfully shy and uneasy I was around him, and how assertive and professional he was around me. In addition to his intellectual strengths, he was handsome. He didn't know it, but I feel in love with him almost instantly, without him knowing.

He would either invite me to lunch or to have a cup of tea in the cafeteria which was a pleasant diversion from my uneasiness because I could concentrate on listening to him talk about his day as a way to avoid talking about mine. We continued to meet on several occasions just to talk. Each time we met, he introduced me to a different blend of tea that he brought to work to share with me during our lunch times. As we sat together more frequently, the kids noticed us. The kids, who I was closer to than others, began to tease us in fun. We would smile sheepishly, and scat them away. Those were good times.

We shared other good times. Riding bikes in the park, feeding the ducks while sitting near the river bank in Bridgewater, Pennsylvania or meeting for lunch at the park in Center Township. I also remember going to movies, shopping for antiques and bargain clothing at Good Will, and sharing his collection of food coupons that really helped to counter the high cost of food. Recalling the best time of all, caused me to smile. It was when I played the lotto for the first time on his dare and won $1,000. We were as excited as young children with money to spend on anything we wanted. I split the winnings 50/50. We filled our refrigerators with all kinds of goodies, bought a couple bottles of wine, and even had enough left over to pay a bill or two, and rent a movie to watch later in the day. Those were good times for sure. I thanked God for the good times, and told myself that there would be more good times ahead.

Then I thought about the goodness of God. After my divorce, I was raising three children by myself. It was tough at times. Helping with homework every night, taking three kids to their extracurricular activities and picking them up, cooking, packing lunches every night, all while working full time during the day. I also decided to return to grad school to obtain a master's in health education and later a PhD. So attending grad school two days a week in the evening was an added responsibility. It was hard, but I made it work with God's help. I was thankful for the faith and grace He had given me to meet every obligation.

Praying and giving thanks for all things were therapeutic, especially during a time like this when I needed to do both. Reading the bible has a way of booting my faith. My favorite inspirational reading of all time comes from Romans 8:28, a promise that rings true for me every day:

And we know that all things work together for good to those who love God, to those who are called according to His purpose.

With this remembrance in mind, I rested on God's word, and I was able to doze off again before seeing the doctor coming around the corner and hearing him say that the surgery was successful. The doctor did come, and his report was bitter sweet. Yes, the surgery was successful, but the fast-growing cancer cells had metastasized to Bruce's lymph nodes in his lower body including his leg bones which explained why he was experiencing bone pain making it more difficult for him to stand or walk.

After surgery, Bruce remained under observation for a while in the recovery room and was wheeled back to his room. Within a few minutes the oncologist entered the room accompanied by the surgeon. The oncology report was positive. The *bone scan* confirmed that the cancer had metastasized to his leg bones and *lymph nodes*. Despite the diagnosis, the doctors were hopeful that Bruce would recover successfully with the help of a *team of specialists* that included the oncologist, orthopedic specialist, neurologist, and dietician, all of whom would work with him as long as needed. The surgeon turned to Bruce with more not-so-good news. He said,

> You will need to undergo another surgery in a couple of days to place rods in both legs that will enable you to walk. Then upon returning home from the hospital, you will also need chemotherapy to kill any lingering cancer cells. *Chemo* is rough. You'll experience some aches and pains, loss of hair in most cases, appetite, weight, and the ability to control urination.[1,2]

Bruce didn't say anything, he just listened. He quickly glanced at the doctor then looked at me. I could see the look of despair in his eyes. He had already been through a lot. The prospect of losing his already thinning hair, additional weight, his appetite, and the ability to control his urination was all too much. The sadness of losing control of his bodily function was plainly visible in the tears that welled up in his eyes, and his silent response gave him the look of one who had resigned himself to die without much struggle.

Today was Monday. His surgery was scheduled for Tuesday, April 22, 2014. I made a reservation to stay at a nearby hotel that night. However, I decided to stay overnight in Bruce's room to be with him. The only accommodation was a recliner chair. That morning I felt stiff and tired from not being able to stretch out like I wanted to. I really needed to get some sleep. A shower and clean clothes would have been appreciated too. Nevertheless, I planned to stay the day and night, but Bruce suggested that I go home, get a shower, make sure the dog was taken care of, secure the house, and come back early tomorrow morning. He probably assumed he would have to stay another day or two post-surgery.

I was about to leave, when one of the nurse's came in to transport Bruce to x-ray. Little did she know that Bruce's sense of humor was still alive and well, despite his feeling poorly. I remember him asking the nurse jokingly, "Do you have any wine? I sure could use a glass or two."

The nurse smiled sheepishly and said, "No sir, I don't, I'm sorry." I just laughed out-loud and shook my head, and hoped she did not take him seriously.

Before leaving, we embraced and gave each other a peck on the cheek. I reminded him that I would be back in the morning long before he goes to surgery.

He said, "Ok. Take my jacket and cane with you when you go."

I replied, "But you will need your coat and cane when I come back to take you home."

"No, I want you to wear the coat. It's a warm coat." he said. I was uncomfortable with his request, but I did what he asked. After I returned home, he called, "Are you home yet."

"Yes, I just got in," I replied.

"Make sure you lock all the doors. In my clothes cupboard is some money. Use it to pay some bills. My credit cards are in the drawer along with the access numbers." he said. I could tell he had just been given a dose of morphine because his speech was slurred.

"Are you ok," I asked.

"I'm ok. I dozed off and thought you were still here. I was talking to you," he said.

"What were you talking about?" I asked.

"I can't' remember," he said. "Oh yea, remember to bring Brandon with you when you come so you won't have to drive back by yourself."

"Ok. Try to get some rest. I will see you early tomorrow. And behave yourself," I said jokingly.

When the Unexpected Occurs

The day of the second surgery had arrived. I woke up around 4:00 am to prepare for the trip back to the hospital. I had just showered when the phone rang. What happened next was a blur. I answered the phone and I heard a man's voice on the other end.

"May I speak to Mrs. Cobb? This is the hospital calling." he said.

I am sure the person introduced himself, but for the life of me I don't remember his name. I knew that it wasn't the doctor, not that it mattered. The news was such a shock that it didn't matter who was the messenger.

"This is she," I said.

"Are you alone?" the voice asked.

I replied, "Yes, I'm getting ready to come there now."

Then he slowly said, "Mrs. Cobb, I am so sorry. Your husband passed early this morning. Some of the cancerous cells had metastasized to his brain. We tried to resuscitate him. He revived for about two minutes then he was gone. I am so sorry."

I heard his voice, but what he said did not register. There was momentary silence. I could not hear what this person was saying to me. Bruce gone? Gone where? What..? I remembered standing over an open drawer and grabbing it to steady myself. I couldn't feel a thing. Still numb, I struggled to collect myself to call his children and mine to let them know what happened. I mechanically struggled to collect myself to call his children and mine to let them know that their father had passed. As I prepared for the trip back to the hospital to view the body and collect Bruce's belongings, I felt like a slow-moving zombie. I think I was in shock.

Brandon, Bruce's son, who lived in Baltimore area, arrived at my home in Philadelphia in almost record time. We rode back to Baltimore together, we were silent the entire trip, we just didn't know what to say. After we arrived, an orderly wheeled Bruce's body to a private area where we could see him. When I pulled the white sheet away from his body to look at his face, he looked as if he was still alive. His skin tone and facial expression had not changed nor the texture of his graying beard. I touched his body; it was cold. It was only then that I realized Bruce was gone. He was not coming back. As I continued to stare at Bruce's body, an official looking person asked me to sign a document releasing Bruce's body so he could be brought back to Pennsylvania for cremation, which is what he wanted. I also signed another document indicating that I was given possession of the few items left in his room.

The drive back to Philadelphia was surreal. I knew Bruce was gone, but when I turned the key in the door and entered the house, a new feeling awaited me. I could still sense Bruce's presence and the loneliness of his absence simultaneously. In his absence a question that still dominates my mind: what was he thinking on the last night before his surgery? I can only imagine what he was thinking. Maybe he knew he was dying and welcomed its coming as freedom. I think maybe he thought about his dreams for his children. Maybe he worried that I would have no one to comfort me during my time of grief. Maybe the pain and morphine mixed together lulled him into thinking about nothing at all. I will never know his final thoughts. But what I do know is that Bruce deeply believed in humanity, and he spent his career for it to be recognized in himself and others.

When Grief Turns Into Reflection

Two years after Bruce passed I decided to sell our home in Philadelphia and move to Atlanta, GA to be close to my daughter and grandson. It's been almost 10 years now since Bruce's passing, and I still reflect on the good times we shared as well as the challenges we faced in coping with erectile dysfunction. As his partner, I was fortunate to have been with Bruce to care for him during the last stretch of his illness.

I remembered him as a man whose condition affected his inability to walk or stand did not keep him from doing what he loved, teaching and counseling students. He never gave up. When he could not stand very long, he used a cane to get around. He continued to teach while sitting on the edge of the desk top in the classroom and counseling students while sitting in his office chair. Teaching, counseling, and helping students seek financial opportunities to advance their education were the joys of his life. Interacting with students motivated him to get up in the morning, get dressed, and go to work.

On work days the staff, who was aware of his work schedule, waited for him to enter the building so they could open the door for him and help him to his office. When he could no longer drive t work because his legs were beginning to swell making it painfully difficult to maneuver the pedals, I would drive him to work. When I pulled up close to the curb outside the building where he worked, I could see the staff waiting at the entrance of the building to open the door for him, and when I arrived to pick him up from work, the staff was positioned to do the same.

Yes, Bruce was gone. On April 22, 2014 he passed away leaving a legacy of not what he did for himself, but what he did for others that would endure for generations to come. Shortly after he passed, Philadelphia Community College and Alvernia University, where he worked full and part-time respectively did a beautiful job organizing memorial services in his honor. The student body, faculty, staff, and community members came together to show their appreciation for the ways in which Bruce enriched their lives. The cards, flowers, well-wishes, and personal testimonies from students and faculty who appreciated Bruce's service, were comforting.

In addition, Alvernia University students, many of whom had taken several of Bruce's courses, later made an additional tribute to Bruce. The students approached the administration and requested that an academic scholarship be established in Bruce's name as a way of giving back and showing their appreciation. I was pleased when the administration requested that I determine the requirements for the scholarship. Receiving such an accolade from students is the most humbling and rewarding experience for an educator. To accept one on behalf of my partner was one of the most fulfilling moments of my life with Bruce.

I would be remiss if I did not express my gratitude for one other thing that might sound strange. Losing Bruce to a disease that took his life too soon is another good thing about losing my husband. I was able to feel the love and caring of my kind neighbors who took time to comfort me in whatever ways they could. I remain so grateful to this day for the outpouring of love and caring from neighbors who stopped by to express their condolences with hugs. Some sent cards along with delicious prepared snacks.

I will never forget my next-door neighbor and dearest friend who would always come by and just sit when I least expected her. Her personality was never quiet. She had a happy go lucky kind of personality that was unpredictable but reassuring. Her kind words, friendly smile, jovial gestures always made me smile. It surely felt so good to chuckle along with her, despite feeling sad. One of the important things I remembered her saying is: Focus on one day at a time. It will be ok. Well, it wasn't ok, not for a long time. I felt stuck, unable to move forward to life by myself. It wasn't until years later, five to be exact, that I found my way back. I didn't understand why I was grieving so hard and for so long when I really wanted relief from it all. My step forward came when I decided to explore my feelings of grief and how I could move pass my feelings to start a new life. I joined a support group whose members I connected with occasionally to express my feelings. I also decided to read as much information as I could about erectile dysfunction so I could help other couples in their struggle with erectile dysfunction.

It has not been an easy journey by no means, but I'm here. I have come a long way. I feel more alive, ready to enjoy a different life from before. I am stronger, more compassionate because of Bruce's death. I seemed to have a new purpose in life, so I joined a couple more self-help groups that were beneficial to my emotional and mental health, such as our community book cub and a congenial group of gym buddies who I see regularly when I go to the gym. To stay connected we committed to meeting for lunch or attending a social activity once per month. I am making more friends, traveling on my own, spending more time getting to know me and what I aspire to do for the remainder of my life. I am discovering the joys and cathartic effects of hurling all my feelings and emotions into writing. This book is my contribution to couples tackling erectile dysfunction together. In addition upon my request, eleven African American men volunteered to share their perceptions of the role of the partner of men dealing with erectile dysfunction. Their genuine desire to "give back" to couples by contributing to this book is remarkable.

CHAPTER 9

The Sexual Partner's Role In Each Phase of Managing Erectile Dysfunction

From A Healthcare Prospective

Two is company three is NOT a crowd.

Erectile dysfunction (ED) is no longer considered a male disorder, but is regarded as a condition of the mind and body for couples. The concept of treating the couple together is increasingly accepted and has become a common practice in many sexual medicine clinics. The importance of the partner's role in assessment of men with ED though well recognized is by no means a universal occurrence. Since the introduction of safe, effective approaches to the management of ED, it has been considered a male medical problem. This attitude leads men with ED being managed in the clinic in isolation of their partners. Most men who seek treatment for erectile dysfunction are in established heterosexual relationships. However, men tend to present in medical settings alone[1], and even when they are invited to bring their partners to the clinic, only a few partners attend. Sexual partners of men with ED have an important role in its management and improvement in quality of sex life; therefore, they should be involved in assessment of, diagnosis, education, counseling, choice of therapy, and rehabilitation.[2-5]

Although each of the following roles of a partner is discussed separately, the partner's myriad roles in men with ED are interconnected and are critical in the management of erectile dysfunction.

Assessment Phase: The Sexual Partner's Role

The partner of the man with ED should volunteer to accompany the man to his initial visit to the primary care physician. The initial visit should include a thorough medical screening including your medical history, a physical examination including examination of genitals for lesions and deformities, a cardiac assessment for hearth health to focus on lipid levels, blood sugar levels (to determine diabetes), and hormonal evaluations including morning serum total testosterone and thyroid function levels. If the physician is comfortable, the physician may administer a sexual and psychological evaluation involving both partners.

The physician may also conduct a sexual and psychological evaluation (similar to a medical intake) that may make conversation around sexual health easier, both with your partner and your doctor.[6] Since it is rarely possible to identify and address all the causes and factors involved in the patient's condition by talking with only one of the partners, the clinician should include the partner who may be able to clarify any discrepancies in the medical history or reveal symptoms of an underlying sexual or medical issue that she or he may be experiencing, which may have some bearing on the patient's ability to achieve or maintain an erection, adequacy and quality of the interest in the relationship.[7]

Once the initial examination is completed, your healthcare provider should be able to determine if other specialists are needed to be involved in your care, such as endocrinologist for hormone issues, a cardiologist for health issues, a neurologist for nerve issues, or a urologist.[8]

Diagnosis: The Sexual Partner's Role

The identification of the nature of erectile dysfunction or suspicion was raised either because of an elevation in your serum prostate-specific antigen (PSA) level or an abnormality of the prostate noted by the digital rectal examination. If the diagnosis is cancer (as discussed in Chapter 4), it is definitely a shock to both you and your partner. Emotions block out any kind of rational thinking much of the time. Feelings of "how can this happen to me?" are normal. After being shocked by the news, additional feelings of self-pity, sadness, and even hopelessness surface, all of which are normal. You may be at a lost as to where to begin to tell those who you know care about you. First start with yourself. Give yourself some time to process and accept what is happening then begin to include those surrounding you, friends, family members, co-workers. If your partner was with you when you received the news, continue to communicate your feelings with your partner.[9,10]

The positive reinforcement of your partner in diagnosis of the problem is invaluable at a time like this when you need it the most. Your partner's supportive attitude, desire to accept and confront ED, and provide hope as you both continue the journey to find a solution are motivating factors that can ease a patient's concerns and bring you and your partner closer together.[11]

Education: The Sexual Partner's Role

Under most circumstances, the partner's attitudes and knowledge of the sexual disorders have a critical role in facilitating men to seek medical help or the issues. A lack of an adequate level of knowledge of male sexual disorders sometimes compels the sexual partner to have a negative response to the development of ED, which might alter the motivation or willingness of the man with ED to seek medical help. For example, the partner might think that ED is not a crucial issue in the couple's personal life or relationship, that the loss of erection is permanent and irreversible, that clinicians are not the right people to help, or that taking drugs to improve erectile function is risky and/or harmful. Inappropriate perspectives or assumptions from the partner can cause men with ED to change their attitude about seeking medical therapy. With comprehensive education and counseling from nurses and others specializing in urology, the pessimistic attitudes of sexual partners toward their partner's ED can change to optimistic.[12,13] However, a negative attitude of a sexual partner can be a source of disappointment causing the man to pull away from his partner and delay much needed medical care.

Choice of Treatment: The Sexual Partner's Role

The involvement of sexual partners in medical intervention of ED is essential. Sexual partners have a critical role in achieving long-term relief of ED after treatment[14] and their attitudes, beliefs, and sexual experience are important in the prognosis of ED. The attitude of men with ED regarding acceptance or rejection of treatment protocols can be changed by their sexual partners.[15]

Sexual partners can support the partner with ED in treatment-seeking through various motivational actions such as talking with each other, showing interest and dealing actively with the problem, appealing to the male self-esteem, supporting the doctor's visit, active cooperation and participation in the treatment and initiating sexual intercourse[16] or other forms of sexual intimacy.

If drug therapy is preferred by the couples, it will have a role in the couple's sexual behavior, as well as affecting the patient's erectile function.[17,18] Most patients with ED consult their clinician in absence of their partners; therefore, active engagement of sexual partners in therapeutic intervention for ED is still a challenge in current clinical practice.[19]

Rehabilitation or Recovery: The Sexual Partner's Role

When clinicians invite both partners to be involved in the discussions on treatment options and modalities to be tried, there is likelihood of increased compliance.[20,21] Sexual recovery is a slow process that requires patience, time, and persistence. Recovery rates area linked to knowledge of couple's sexual needs in the relationship. Partner's attendance at the clinic is also important so that she/he can learn about the medical intervention recommended and how and when it should be used.

Research indicates that in general, sharing any intervention early may lead to better recovery of erectile function.[22] Because the effectiveness of interventions usually are not obtained overnight, the patient and his sexual partner should not expect immediate results. Sexual recovery takes time and depending on the importance the sexual partner and partner with ED puts on sexual intercourse, sexual recovery can be prolonged. For example, a sexual partner may be less interested in helping the man achieve sexual intercourse iffy interested in this activity. She/he might be reluctant to offer adequate sexual stimulation and positive reinforcement feedback, an important consideration when the man uses a treatment that requires sexual stimulation for its full effect (for example sildenafil and apomorphine.[22-23]

Partners may also be less enthusiastic in providing stimulation if they feel that they are unlikely to get out of the sexual interaction what they really would and what is important for them in contributing to their sexual satisfaction and recovery. Although a man with ED seeks a means to have an erection to enable him to have sexual intercourse, his partner may have a totally different agenda.[24] So when given the opportunity to share feelings, it is the role of the sexual partner to be transparent and honest about their feelings and attitudes toward sexual function and the recovery of sexual intercourse.

Partners can also assist men with ED by becoming involved in the actual treatment process, which appears to improve compliance and recovery. Partners' can express the feeling that they want to be involved in the initiation of their partner's erection. When a man has a medical drug induced erection, such as intracavernosal injection therapy, his partner may have feelings of resentment that the erection was achieved without her/his involvement, and such feelings lead to the partner to consider the erection process as unnatural. The role of the partner may be something simple as in the case of intracavernosal injection therapy, she/he may do anything from opening the pack to actually giving the injection,[24] after given directions on how to carefully insert the needle in the penis.

Other ways in which sexual partners can invest in the recovery process is by preparing nutritious meals, doing prescribed exercises with your partner, continuing going to doctor's visits, encouraging your partner to be patient because you are, and spending quality time gently touching and caressing him in places that he indicates are comfortable for you to do so.

Although erectile dysfunction is the inability to attain or maintain an erection in the male, it is a problem that affects those around him, especially his sexual partner. Sexual problems and relationship conflict are common in partners dealing with ED, that can negatively affect the process of managing ED. Problems with relationships maybe psychological or physical but unless she/he is assessed along with the man who is experiencing ED, the problem(s) will go unrecognized and the patient's prognosis in terms of re-establishing satisfying intercourse will be compromised. It is unfortunate that many clinical environments are not conducive to partner attendance.[25]

If this is the case, my advice: find another urologist whose clinic will welcome the partner's involvement. Bruce and I were fortunate to have visited our urologist, Dr. Author Burnett, who welcomed and encouraged me to be involved in all stages of the management of my husband's erectile dysfunction. I am confident that in your role as partner to a man with ED that you will be an active participant in securing a clinician who is conducive to partner presence.

This chapter focused on the partner's role in managing erectile dysfunction from a healthcare provider's point of view. The emphasis healthcare providers place on good communication and cooperation between partners, their sexual partner, and their clinicians are very important for achieving good treatment outcomes.[26] However, the opinions of men with ED are equally important when it comes to their perspectives of their partner's role in management of sexual dysfunction. In the next chapter the partner's role is described from the perspective of eleven men of color, mostly African American. The men with ED discuss how a partner's attitudes, behaviors, and values related to ED can affect a couple's relationship and the man's desire to seek help in managing erectile issues.

CHAPTER 10

The Sexual Partner's Role in ED

From the Perspective of Eleven Men of Color

Giving back.

This chapter is limited to a description of eleven men's perception of their partner's role in dealing with erectile dysfunction, either as past recollection or current descriptions. The men who volunteered to share their perceptions of the role of their partner in coping with ED expected to be supported. Most received support from partners, a few others did not. Most of the men were married or divorced. A couple men never married, but provided their opinions in the absence of marriage. Their ages ranged from 39-73 years. Most men identified themselves as Black or African American. One man wanted to be identified as Haitian.

The purpose of inviting men to share their experiences was twofold: (1) to give voice to the eleven men who wanted to pay homage to men, despite their varied experiences with their partners, and (2) to not to generalize, but to provide a thumb nail sketch of the multi-dimensional roles partners may play in determining whether the man would seek diagnosis and treatment for their ED. The quotes included in this section are the views expressed by the men in response to the question, how do you perceive the role of partners who are in relationships with men coping with erective dysfunction?

When most men noticed their initial changes in erectile function, they did not initially talk about their inability to achieve or maintain an erection. They considered the topic of erectile dysfunction to be off-limits to their partners. However, men whose partners were willing to engage in open and honest communication, became less concerned about being rejected, despite their inability to achieve or maintain an erection.

Two men, who never married, were not experiencing erectile issues expressed their views about the role of the partner if they were to marry. They believed that being open and honest were hallmark characteristics of a supportive partner.

> Although I don't have a partner, I would want her to be open to what I was feeling, and to work with me to get the help needed when the time comes. If she was mean and not supportive, I would hesitate to open up to her because of the way she hurt me.

> I'm not concerned about myself. What I may go through when my time comes is not that important. If I were married, my job is to please her in any way I can. If she is going through some things, I want to help her. If I am going through some things, I'll be honest with her too. This is how she supports me, and I support her.

Another man who was married at the time of the interview, but single when he was experiencing erectile concerns while taking care of his mother who was terminally ill with dementia. As the caretaker and only child, he associated his erectile changes to the stress of taking care of his mom. He indicated that his intimate partners (at the time he had more than one) were supportive in their understanding of what he was going through and the effects of stress on the body and mind.

> I remember that my penis could not get erect. At first I was in denial. I had two girlfriends, who were nurses so they both knew what I was going through. One recommended Xanax to alleviate stress, but I didn't take it. In the end, being a spiritual person, I just depended on God more so than a partner to get me through.

Taking the Pressure Off

Two other men referred to the phrase "taking the pressure off," to describe the role of a partner in relieving the man from being responsible for satisfying his partner through coitus or sexual intercourse. When partners of men with ED suggested others ways to satisfy them sexually, such as oral sex or use of a vibrator, men with ED viewed their partners as advocates or leaders which to them reinforced their manhood and caused them to seek help.

> When a man is loved, he feels respected. When a partner is empathetic or can just imagine what a man goes through, that's respect to me. A partner can "take the pressure off" and

be the advocate or leader in convincing the man that this sexual performance is not the only thing that defines him as a man.

It is very important to have a supportive partner. I would rather be with someone than to be by myself because a caring partner will help you figure it out. It's a partner problem, I mean finding a solution. We can't figure it out by ourselves. A partner can help by being the first to encourage a man by "taking the pressure off." It's not what a man can't do, it's what he can do that counts. My partner wanted to understand what was happening, but showed little feeling or interest in having sex. She never really discussed what was happening. To her it was no big deal, but it was important to me. I'm satisfied because I am fixed now. I was broken, but now I am fixed (chuckles to himself). Having the inflatable penile implant was the best thing I could do for my situation. I can go as long as I want (chuckle).

When Both Partners Provide Positive Reinforcement

Another man had sickle cell disease (SCD). Unlike healthy blood cells that are smooth, round, bendable and can easily flow through blood vessels and carry oxygen to every part of the body, sickled cells are irregular-shaped and do not carry oxygen well, which can result in diminished oxygen delivery to organs causing sexual dysfunction and cause other complications **Figure 7** (page 39).

Because his partner learned how to be supportive which led to his willingness to seek help, the next man's experience was starkly different from the previous man's experience. Keeping sexual intimacy alive within a relationship requires positive reinforcing feedback from one partner to another, especially at the onset of ED. Initially, the sexual partner may feel both guilty thinking she is the problem and that the man with ED does not love her. Communication is key. He considered his partner an attribute rather than a liability.

> My partner noticed the changes. I noticed her frustration and had to say something. At first she thought it was her, but I told her that it was me and not her. I think ladies need to respect a man who is experiencing erectile dysfunction and imagine what the man is going through. I think love is respect. My partner definitely understands my difficulty. She knows that a man's sexual performance cannot be the only thing that defines a man. She was really affirming and an asset to me as far as my sexual function is concerned.

When the Partner Is Secure

Experiencing erectile dysfunction is tough. It can be devastating to couples, but for several men, who had confident and supportive partners, these three men were able to cope with their erection changes in way that was beneficial. A confident partner who is not afraid to communicate in a positive manner was a form of "healing" that caused them to openly talk about the changes and seek treatment.

When my partner is confident and willing to step outside herself to talk openly about her sexual experience with me, whether the experience was good or bad, it's kind of healing. It's encouraging and makes men want to get help.

I want someone with confidence to talk about my performance. Talking to my partner about what's happening was encouraging and caused me to get help.

A good partner can heal a man if she is confident and secure with the man. Her words of encouragement can heal a man and cause him to get help.

One other man went into detail about what he was experiencing including his partner's reaction to his erectile changes. When he started experiencing excruciating pain and the inability to urinate regularly, he refused to go to the doctor because he was afraid that the diagnosis would be cancer. Instead he turned to his older sister who offered her non-judgmental support. When the pain became unbearable, his sister convinced him to go see his doctor. In fact, she accompanied him to the doctor and even gave him some encouraging advice—"man up, you'll be ok."

After several tests, the doctor recommended venous and arterial surgery to alleviate the painful urination. While the surgery solved his urinary problem on one hand, it effected his reproductive function. Without getting into much detail which he could not recall at the time of the interview, he said the surgery left him without the ability to produce semen which meant he could not have children. As an older man, he wasn't concerned about his inability to have children. However, he wondered how his new found intimate relationship with his lady friend would react to the news.

I did tell her about the surgery and what I had experienced prior to surgery. When I told her I couldn't produce semen or have kids, her response was…really…wow! She told me not to worry, and that it would be ok. She asked me if I could have an erection, and I told her yes, no problem in that area. Her response just built my confidence. In fact, she was happy that I went with the surgery. So to me, she was very positive. She made me feel confident in my sexuality. We are still in love, still friends. My sister was a big help too. Having a supportive partner is very important.

The power of a supportive partner whether a caring relative or an intimate sexual partner is undeniably an asset to encouraging men with ED to seek help, despite their interadaption. However, when men don't have supportive intimate partners, the inability to achieve or maintain an erection is most likely to carry the added weights of discouragement and defeat.

When the Sexual Partner's Initial Reaction Is Negative

One man had Multiple Sclerosis. Multiple Sclerosis can affect a man or woman. It's a condition that affects the brain, spinal cord, nervous system, and sexual function. He felt his partner did not encourage him to talk about his inability to achieve an erection. Instead, he felt his only recourse was to shut down.

I remember when I first had a problem. My partner got very frustrated and told me to get off of her. That really hurt my ego. I said ok, and I apologized and told her that this never happened before. I would have preferred if she was the advocate, meaning someone who can take the lead in encouraging the man to try something else or try again later on. But that didn't happen.

Another man considered having his partner's respect essential to his manhood and self-esteem. However, when his partner's reaction was not what he expected, her reaction left him feeling hurt and uncertain of his sexual ability even after he sought effective treatment.

It was devastating to me. I never talked about it to her because I didn't know how to start the conversation without it ending up in an argument. I woke up one morning and I wanted to have sex. She seemed all right with that. When I tried to put it in, it just went soft. I tried over and over hoping it would get hard, but it wouldn't work. She blew out a sigh of air that made me feel like she was relieved or glad it was over.

Did you question her about what she was feeing at that moment? I asked during the interview.

Yes, I did ask her what did that mean. She never really answered. She just said when you can do something, let me know. After that, I just left her alone for a long time because my ego and self-confidence in my ability to please her were crushed, I guess. Since then I'm ok now. I did go get checked out and I got help. In fact, after thinking about it for a long time, I went with the implant, the inflatable kind. Even though she did go to the doctor's with me, I still felt the damage was done. I kind of wished she didn't go. It took a long time for me to respect myself as a man after that because I was really hurt and felt disrespected by what she said, but I stayed in the relationship.

Having a sexual partner who is respectful, understanding, and willing to communicate about their reaction to a man's inability to have an erection are qualities men desire in a partner. In closing, one man said it best,

My partner just made excuses, like 'I have to get up early in the morning,' which made me feel that she was not interested in me. Talking is important. Taking the time to at least try to be intimate is important too. Women need to be respectful and understand that men have feelings too.

Summary

This chapter presented the role of the sexual partner in managing erectile dysfunction. findings of an interview with nine African American men between the ages of 39-73 years who for the most part experienced changes in erectile function, and changes in emotions depending on the initial reaction of their sexual partner. The combined influence of biological, psychological, and beliefs on women's behaviors and responses to their partners' erectile changes resulted in the identification of what men with ED considered were important attributes of a partner. The act of relying on their sexual partner to be supportive, understanding, sensitive to a man's loss of manhood, willing to learn, and respectful, the most acceptable way for a man with ED and his partner to cope with unpredictable erectile changes, is a practice that became difficult for men with ED who were experiencing a wide range of physical and emotional changes due to uncertainty and fear. Having a supportive partner can be effective in improving the management, care, quality of sex life, and therefore, should be invited into every phase of the journey to finding a solution for erectile dysfunction.

CHAPTER 11

Lessons Learned

Reflections.

I t's been almost 8 years since Bruce passed, and I still struggle sometime to make sense of it all. I am grateful for the serenity prayer I learned long ago that's so applicable when experiencing life-changing events, "God grant me the serenity to accept the things I cannot change, courage to change the things I can, and wisdom to know the difference." Life goes on, as the saying goes. I continue to praise and thank God in all things. I continue to live and enjoy every moment that includes writing about what interests me, going the gym, traveling here and there, and spending time with family and friends. I'm so grateful for the support of family and friends. I have been blessed so much through this experience.

Delaying Visiting Your Urologist Will Not Solve the Problem

If there are two lessons I learned from this experience. The first lesson is captured in the words of Benjamin Franklin, "don't put off until tomorrow what you can do today." This saying is especially applicable to seeking treatment for erectile dysfunction. Yes, it is true in most cases that couples do have time to make a plan of action for coping with ED. However, the plan does not include procrastinating. Be intentional about communicating with your partner, seeing the urologist for diagnosis, asking questions, and discussing treatment options. The partner's involvement in all phases of the journey to finding a solution for ED may prove to be critical to a man's psychological and physical well-being and to the restoration of sexual intimacy.

The Importance of Keeping the Faith

The second lesson I learned is to keep the faith. Having faith in God played a very strong role throughout this experience including my interaction with family members. I wanted them to see God in this experience, and in me. I have a message for all men and their partners who are experiencing erectile dysfunction or any life-changing event for that matter.

What matters the most is your steadfast faith in God from the beginning to the end of the journey. Trusting and believing that "all things work together for good for those who love God and who are called according to his purpose" is no easy task when you don't know for sure what the outcome is going to be. I want to go on record saying that I have no regrets. I thank God for allowing me to love a man who took pride in serving others. I have no regrets about employing Dr. Bud Burnett as our urologist. I remain confident in his superior expertise, his caring, and personal ethics in providing the best evidence-based therapies when it comes to male sexual health. He is a trusted authority. More importantly, the God I serve did not let me down. He said he would not leave me or forsake me, and he's kept his promise. I am so thankful to know that HE was there in the trenches with me. Without faith, I would not have had the strength to get through the difficult days of adjusting to not having a partner. Without faith I would not have the motivation to write this book as an inspiration to other couples who are experiencing erectile dysfunction.

Life Goes On

So what's next on the horizon for me? I plan to continue to write perhaps a second book based on the eleven men's perceptions of erectile dysfunction including their management of erectile changes, sociocultural influences, spiritual factors that influenced their perceptions of their erectile function experiences, all of which is not a part of this book but was included in the initial interview. In concordance, I am developing a 4-week on-line course for singles and couples on how to cope with erectile dysfunction, with a special focus on the role of partners of men with erectile dysfunction.

Furthermore, I continue to be interested in providing support to men and families affected by erectile dysfunction. To that end, I contacted ZERO- the End of Prostate Cancer, a nonprofit organization that provides support services to family and community members impacted by prostate cancer as well as training for individuals who are interested in becoming support group leaders. Being a part of an organization with the mission to end prostate cancer is a wonderful way to help all who are in most need.

Summary and Conclusion

Erectile dysfunction is no longer a male disorder, a condition men should have to experience alone. Clinicians have an important role in approaching a taboo subject that used to be viewed solely as a result of a physical problem that many men prefer to manage on their own without the support of a partner. Clinicians also know that a supportive sexual partner to a man with ED can be a valuable asset in the management of erectile dysfunction. Despite the many taboos that overshadow men's sexual prowess and self-esteem, they, like partners world-wide, can be a source of strength and encouragement to men with ED, which more importantly can lead to support in assessment, diagnosis, and effective treatment and restoration of sexual intimacy. It is my hope that this guide for couples who are experiencing erectile dysfunction will promote the healthcare of all men during a time in their life when they need it the most.

Endnotes

CHAPTER I:
Creating a Safe Place For Partners to Communicate

1. Moss R. Advice for women on how to deal with your partner's erectile dysfunction. Accessed September 12, 2022, https://www.huffintonpost.co.uk/2016.02/03 how-erectile-dysfunction-affects-women_n_9149362.hlml. Accessed December 12, 2022

2. Burnett AL. (2021, October 27). The stigma of depreciating manhood in men with sexual dysfunction [video]. YouTube, www.urologytimes.com/view/the-stigma-of-depreciating-manhood-in-men-with-sexual-dysfunction. Accessed December 12, 2022.

3. Sritof S. (2022, May 24). What to do if your partner has lost interest in sex. Verywellmind.https://www.verywellmind.com/partner-not-interested-in-sex-397053. Accessed December 12, 2022.

4. Approaching erectile dysfunction: the woman's perspective. www.totalnutritionandtherapeutics.com/approaching-erectile-dysfunction-the-womans-perspective. Accessed December 12, 2022.

CHAPTER 2
Male Reproductive Anatomy

1. Burnett AL. *The Manhood Rx Every Man's Guide to Improve Sexual Health and Overall Wellness*: Rowan & Littlefield Publishing Group: Lanham, Maryland, 2023, pp 12-18.

2. King BM. (2021). Average size erect penis: fiction, fact, and the need for counseling, Journal of Sex and Marital Therapy, 47; 1, 80-89 DOI: 10.1080/0092623x.2020. 1787279. Accessed December 12, 2023.

3. Alexander LL, LaRosa JH, Bader H, Garfield S, Alexander WJ. (2020) 8th ed. Jones & Bartlett: Burlington, MA. pp 78-81.

4. Ellsworth P. Complications and Treatment: What is erectile dysfunction (ED), and what happens if I have ED after treatment for my prostate cancer. In *100 Questions & Answers About Prostate Cancer* (5th ed., pp.179-194). Jones & Bartlett: Burlington, MA. 2019.

CHAPTER 3
Human Sexual Response

1. Burnett AL. *The Manhood Rx Every Man's Guide to Improve Sexual Health and Overall Wellness*: Rowan & Littlefield Publishing Group: Lanham, Maryland, 2023, pp 21-26.

CHAPTER 4
Symptoms, Causes, and Risk Factors of Erectile Dysfunction

1. Erectile Dysfunction. Information posted by Cleveland Clinic. https://my.clevelandclinic.org/health/diseases/10035-erectile-dysfunction#symptoms-and-causes. Accessed December 12, 2022.

2. Erectile Dysfunction. Information posted by Johns Hopkins Medical School. https://www.hopkinsmedicine.org/health/conditions-and-diseases/erectile-dysfunction. Accessed December 12, 2022

3. Erectile Dysfunction. Information posted by Johns Hopkins Medical School.https://www.hopkinsmedicine.org/health/conditions-and-diseases/erectile-dysfunction. Accessed December 12, 2022

4. Some drugs may cause your erectile dysfunction. Harvard Heath Publishing: Harvard Medical School. https://www.health.harvard.edu/mens-health/ some-drugs-may-cause-your-erectile-dysfunction. Accessed December 12, 2022.

5. Javaron V., Neves, M. Erectile dysfunction and hypertension: impact on cardiovascular risk and treatment. *International Journal of Hypertension* (2012, May 9). Published online 10.1155/2012/627278.

6. What is venous leakage and how does it cause erectile dysfunction (ED)? Retrieved September 12, 2022 from International Society for Sexual Medicine Website.https://www.issm.info/sexual-health-qa/what-is-venous-leakage-and-how-does-it-cause-erectile-dysfunction-ed Accessed December 12, 2022.

7. Neelima V, Edlelman S. (2001). Diabetes and Erectile Dysfunction. *Clinical Diabetes*, 19 (1), 45-47. Accessed September 12, 2022. https://diabetesjournals.org/clinical/article/19/1/45/217/Diabetes-and-Erectile-Dysfunction. Accessed December 12, 2022.

8. Sexual relations in kidney failure for men. National Kidney Foundation. Retrieved September 12, 2022 from National Foundation Kidney Foundation Web site https://www.kidney.org.uk/sexual-relationship-in-kidney-failure-for-men Accessed December 12, 2022.

9. Valeo T. Biking and erectile dysfunction: a real risk? Retrieved September 12, 2022 from WebMD Web site. Reviewed by Michael W. Smith, MD on September 2007.https://www.webmd.com/men/features/biking-and-erectile-dysfunction-a-real-risk. Accessed December 12, 2022.

CHAPTER 5
Current Treatment Options

1. Karaks, S., Burnett, A. L.. The medical and surgical treatment of erectile dysfunction: a review and update, *The Canadian Journal of Urology*™. International Supplement 2020: 28-35. https://www.canjurol.com/html/free-articles/Cdn_JU27-S3_09_DrBurnett_S.pdf. Accessed December 12, 2022.

2. Hatzimouratidis K, Salonia A, Adaikan G et al. Pharmacotherapy for erectile dysfunction: recommendations from the Fourth International Consultation for Sexual Medicine (ICSM) 2015. *Journal of Sexual Medicine* 2016; 13(4):465-488.

3. Hatzimouratidis K, Hatzichristou DG. A comparative review of the options for treatment of erectile dysfunction; Which treatment for which patient? *Drugs* 2005;65(12):1621-1650.

4. Limoncin E, Gravina GL, Corona G et al. Erectile function recovery in men treated with phosphodiesterase type 5 inhibitor administration after bilateral nerve-sparing radical prostatectomy; A systematic review of placebo-controlled randomized trials with trial sequential analysis. *Andrology* 2017; 5(5):863-872.

5. Yang L, Qian S, Liu L et al. Phosphodiesterase-5 inhibitors could be efficacious in the treatment of erectile dysfunction after radiotherapy for prostate cancer: A systematic review and meta-analysis. *Urology International* 2013;90(3):339-341.

6. Vardi M, Nini A. Phosphodiesterase inhibitors for erectile dysfunction in patients with diabetes mellitus. *Cochrane Database System* Review 2007;CD002187.

7. Liao X, Qui S, Bao Y, Wanh, W, Wang L, Wei Q. Comparative efficacy and safety of phosphodiesterase type 5 inhibitors for erectile dysfunction in diabetic men.; A Bayesian network meta-analysis of randomized controlled trials. *World Journal of Urology* 2019;37(6):1061-1074.

8. Burnett, AL. Nitric Oxide in the Penis: Physiology and Pathology. *The Journal of Urology* 1997;157(1):320-324.

9. Karaks, S., Burnett, A. L. The medical and surgical treatment of erectile dysfunction: a review and update, *The Canadian Journal of Urology*™. International Supplement; 2020; 28-35.

10. Shabsigh R, Kaufman JM, Steidle C, Padma-Nathan H. Randomized study of testosterone gel as adjunctive therapy to siddenafil in hypogonadal men with erectile dysfunction who do not respond to sildenafil alone. *Journal of Urology* 2004; 172(2):658-663.

11. Buvat J, Montoral F, Maggi M et al. Hypogonadal men nonresponders to the PDE5 inhibitor tadalafil benefit from normalization of testosterone levels with a 1% hydroalcoholic testosterone gelin the treatment of erectile dysfunction (TADTEST study). *Journal of Sexual Medicine* 2011;8(1):284-293.

12. Price DE, Cooksey G, Jehu D, Bentley, S, Hearnshaw, JR, Osborn DE. The management of impotence in diabetic men by vacuum tumescence therapy. *Diabetic Medicine* 1991;8(10): 964-967.

13. Lee M, Sharifi R. Non-invasive management options for erectile dysfunction when phosphodiesterase type 5 inhibitor fails. *Drugs Aging* 2018;35(3):175-187.

14. Liu C, Lopez DS, Chen M,Wang R. Penile rehabilitation therapy following radical prostatectomy: a meta-analysis. *Journal of Sexual Medicine* 2017;14(12):1496-1503.

15. Levine, L. A., Dimitriou, R. J. Vacuum constriction and external erection devices in erectile dysfunction. *Urology Clinics of North American*, 2001;28(2):335-341.

16. Ellsworth, P. Complications and Treatment: What is erectile dysfunction (ED), and what happens if I have ED after treatment for my prostate cancer. In *100 Questions & Answers About Prostate Cancer* (5th ed., pp.179-194). Jones & Bartlett, 2019.

17. Karakus, S, Burnett A. L. The medical and surgical treatment of erectile dysfunction: a review and update, *The Canadian Journal of Urology* International;2020;27(Suppl 3):28-35.

18. Harin P-N, Hellstrom W JG, Kaiser FE, Labasky RF, et al. for the Medicated Urethral System for Erection (MUSE) Study Group. *The New England Journal of Medicine*, 1997;336:1-7.

19. Ellsworth, P. Complications and Treatment: In *100 Questions & Answers About Prostate Cancer* (5th ed., pp.179-194). Jones & Bartlett,2019.

20. Belew, D., Klassen, Z., Lewis, R. W. Intracavernosal injection for the diagnosis, evaluation, and treatment of erectile dysfunction: a review, *Sexual Medicines Review*, 2015, 3(1):11-23.

21. Heaton JP, Lording D, Liu SN et al. Intracavernosal alprostadil is effective for the treatment of erectile dysfunction in diabetic men. *Journal of Impotence Research*, 2002;3(1):11-23.

22. Burnett, A. L., Nehra, A., Breau, R. H.,et al. Erectile dysfunction: AUA Guideline. *Journal of Urology*, 2018, 200(3), 633-641.

23. Karakus, S., Burnett, A. L. The medical and surgical treatment of erectile dysfunction: a review and update, *The Canadian Journal of Urology*™. International Supplement: 2020, 28-35.

24. Ellsworth, P. Complications and Treatment: In *100 Questions & Answers About Prostate Cancer* (5th ed., pp.179-194). Jones & Bartlett,2019.

25. Dick B, Tsambarlis P, Reddy A, Hellstrom WJ. An update on:long-term outcomes of penile prosthesis for the treatment of erectile dysfunction. *Experimental Review of Medical Devices* 2019;16(4);281-286.

26. Burnett AL, Nehra A, Breau RH et al. Erectile dysfunction:AUA Guideline. *Journal of Urology* 2018;200(3):633-641.

27. Karakus, S, Burnett A. L. The medical and surgical treatment of erectile dysfunction: a review and update, *The Canadian Journal of Urology* International; 2020;27(Suppl 3):28-35.

28. Caplan, A.L., Correa, D. The MSC: an injury drugstore. *Cell Stem Cell*, 2011, 9(1), 11-15.

29. Qiu, X., Sun, C., Yu,W. et al. Combined strategy of mesenchymal stem cell injection with vascular endothelial growth factor gene therapy for treatment of diabetes-associated erectile dysfunction. *Journal of Andrology*, 2012, 33(1), 37-44.

30. Ning, H., Liu, G., Lin, G., Yang, R., Lue, T. F., Lin, C. S. Fibroblast growth factor 2 promotes endothelial differentiation of adipose tissue-derived stem cells. *Journal of Sexual Medicine*, 2009, 6(4), 967-979.

31. Kim, I. G., Piao, S., Lee, J. Y. Effect of an adipose-derived stem cell and nerve growth factor-incorporated hydrogel on recovery of erectile function in a rat model of cavernous nerve. *Tissue Engineering Part A*, 2013;19(1-2), 14-23.

32. Yiou R, Hamidou L, Bire B et al. Safety of intercavernous bone marrow-mononuclear cells for postradical prostatectomy erectile dysfunction; an open dose-escalation pilot study. *European Urology* 2016;69(6);988-991.

33. Levy JA, Marchand M, Iorio L et al. Determining the feasibility of managing erectile dysfunction in humans with placentalderived stem cells. *Journal of Osteopath Association* 2016;116(1):e1-5.

34. Vardi Y, Appel B, Kilchevsky A et al. Does low intensity extracorporeal shock wave therapy have a physiological effect on erectile dysfunction? Short-term results of a randomized, double-blind, sham controlled study. *Journal of Urology* 2012;187(5):1769-1775.

35. Kitrey ND, Gruenwald I, Appel B et al. Penile low-intensity shockwave treatment is able to shift PDE5i nonresponders to responders: a double-blind, sham controlled study. *Journal of Urology* 2016;195(5):1550-1555.

36. Vardi Y, Appel B, Jacib G et al. Can low-intensity extracorporeal shockwave therapy improve erectile function? A 6-month follow-up pilot study in patients with organic erectile dysfunction. *European Urology* 2010;58(2):243-248.

37. Karakus, S, Burnett A. L. The medical and surgical treatment of erectile dysfunction: a review and update, *The Canadian Journal of Urology* International;2020;27(Suppl 3):28-35.

38. Scott, S., Roberts, M., Chung, E. Platelet-rich plasma and treatment of erectile dysfunction: critical review of literature and global trends in platelet-rich plasma clinics. *Sexual Medicine Reviews*, 2019;7(2): 306-312.

39. Matz, E. L., Pearlman, A. M., Terlecki, R. P. Safety and feasibility of platelet-rich fibrin matrix injections for treatment of common urologic conditions, *Investigative Clinical Urology*, 2018, 59,(1), 61-65.

40. Epifanova, M. V., Chaylyi, M. E., Krasnov, A. O. Investigation of mechanisms of action of growth factors of autologous platelet-rich plasma used to treat erectile dysfunction. *Urologiia Urology*, 2017, 4, 46-48.

41. Epifanova, M., V., Gvasalia, B. R., Durashov, M. A., et al. Platelet-rich plasma therapy for male sexual dysfunction myth or reality? *Sexual Medicine Reviews*, 2020, 8(1), 106-113.

42. Campbell, J. D.,Burnett, A. L. Neuroptotective and nerve regenerative approaches for treatment of erectile dysfunction after cavernous nerve injury, *International Journal of Molecular Science*, 2017, 18(8), 1794.

43. Karakus, S, Burnett A. L. The medical and surgical treatment of erectile dysfunction: a review and update, *The Canadian Journal of Urology* International;2020;27(Suppl 3):28-35.

CHAPTER 6
The Initial Diagnosis

1. Burnett, AL. Nitric Oxide in the Penis: *Physiology and Pathology. The Journal of Beling.*

2. Burnett, AL. *The Manhood Rx Every Man's Guide to Improve Sexual Health and Overall Wellness*: Rowan & Littlefield: Lanham, MD. 2023.

CHAPTER 7
The Second Diagnosis

1. Burnett, AL. Patients Guide to Prostate Cancer. Massachusetts: Jones & Bartlett. 2011.

2. Chemotherapy: Types & How They Work - Cleveland Clinic my.clevelandclinic.org/health/treatments/16859-chemotherapy

3. American Cancer Society. Cancer facts for men. https://www.cancer.org/healthy/cancer-facts/cancer-facts-for-men.html (assessed April 9, 2022).

4. Hara, M, Inorre, T, Fukuyama, T. Some physiochemical characteristics of gamma-seminoprotein, an antigenic component specific for human seminal plasma. *Japanese Journal of Legal Medicine* 1971; 25: 322-324.

5. Li, TS. Beling, CG. Isolation and characterization of two specific antigens of human seminal plasma. Fertility and Sterilization; 1973 February 24(2):134-144.

6. Sensabaugh, GF. Isolation and characterization of a men-specific protein from human seminal plasma: a potential new marker for semen identification. *Journal of Forensic Science* 1978; 23(1):106-115.

7. Graves, HC. Sensabaugh, GF, Blake ET. Postcoital detection of a male-specific semen protein. Application to the investigation of rape. *New England Journal of Medicine*; 1985 February 7. 312(6):338-343.

8. Goetz, T, Burnett, AL. Prostate cancer risk after anti-androgen treatment for priapism. *International Urology and Nephrology*; 2014 April 46(4):757-760.

9. Burnett, AL. *The Manhood Rx Every Man's Guide to Improve Sexual Health and Overall Wellness*: Rowan & Littlefield: Lanham, MD. 2023.

10. Acute Ishemic Priapism: an AUA/SMSNA Guideline. Journal of Urology; November 2021. https//doi.org/10:1097/Ju.0000000000002236.

CHAPTER 8
The Day of Surgery

1. American Cancer Society. Chemotherapy Side Effects. (https://www.cancer.org/treatment/treatments-and-side-effects/treatment-types/chemotherapy/chemotherapy-side-effects.html) Accessed 10/20/2022.

2. Chemotherapy: Types & How They Work - Cleveland Clinic my.clevelandclinic.org/health/treatments/16859-chemotherapy

CHAPTER 9
The Sexual Partner's Role in Each
Phase of Managing Erectile Dysfunction

1. Barnes T. Female partners in erectile dysfunction: what is her position? *Journal of Sexual Marital Therapy* 1998;13:233-240.

2. Riley A. The role of the partner in erectile dysfunction and its treatment. *International Journal of Impotence Research* 2002;Suppl 1, S105-S109, DOI: 10.1038/sj/ijir/3900800.

3. Carvalheira AA, Piera NM, Maroco J, Forjaz V. Dropout in the treatment of erectile dysfunction with PDE5: a study on prediction and a qualitative analysis of reasons for discontinuation. *Journal of Sexual Medicine* 2012, 9, 2361-2369.

4. Melman A et al. Psychosocial issues in diagnosis and treatment. In: Jardin A et al. (eds). Erectile dysfunction: *First International Consultation on Erectile Dysfunction*, July 1999. Paris. Health Publishers Ltd: Plymouth, 2000, pp 407-436.

5. Dorey G. Partners 2001. perspectives of erectile dysfunction: literature review, *British Journal of Nursing* 10,187-195.

6. Burnett, AL. *The Manhood Rx Every Man's Guide to Improve Sexual Health and Overall Wellness*: Rowan & Littlefield, Lanham, Boulder, New York & London, 2023.

7. Riley A. The role of the partner in erectile dysfunction and its treatment. *International Journal of Impotence Research* 2002;Suppl 1, S105-S109, DOI: 10.1038/sj/ijir/3900800.

8. Burnett, AL. *The Manhood Rx Every Man's Guide to Improve Sexual Health and Overall Wellness*: Rowan & Littlefield, Lanham, Boulder, New York & London, 2023.

9. Burnett, AL. *Patients Guide to Prostate Cancer*. Massachusetts: Jones & Bartlett. 2011.

10. Burnett, AL. *The Manhood Rx Every Man's Guide to Improve Sexual Health and Overall Wellness*: Rowan & Littlefield, Lanham, Boulder, New York & London, 2023.

11. Impotence Imposes on Relationships - Erectile Dysfunction – WebMD www.com/erectile-dysfunction/features/ impotence-imposes-on-relationships

12. Hongjiun Li, Gao T, Wang R. The role of the sexual partner in managing erectile dysfunction 2016; 13, 168 *Nature Reviews Urology*, 168-177.

13. Fisher WA et al. Communication about erectile dysfunction among men with ED, partners of men with ED; and physicians: the Strike Up a Conversation Study (Part II) Journal of Men's Health Gender 2, 64-78 (2005).

14. Dean J et al. Integrating partners into erectile dysfunction treatment: Improving the sexual experience for the couple *International Journal of Clinical Practice* 62, 127-133 (2008).

15. Fisher W et al. Eardley I, McCabe M, Erectile dysfunction (Ed) is as shared sexual concern of couples II: association of female partner characteristics with male partner characteristics with male partner ED seeking treatment and phosphodiesterase type 5 inhibitor. *Journal of Sexual Medicine* 6, 3111-3124 (2009).

16. Gerster S, Gunzler, C, Roesler, Leiber C, Berner MM. Treatment motivation of men with ED: what motivates en wit ED to seek professional help and how can women support their partners? *International Journal of Impotence Research* 2013 25(2): 56-62. DOI: 10.1038/ijir.2012.37. Epub 2012 Oct 11.

17. Fisher W et al. Eardley I, McCabe M, Erectile dysfunction (Ed) is as shared sexual concern of couples II: association of female partner characteristics with male partner characteristics with male partner ED seeking treatment and phosphodiesterase type 5 inhibitor. *Journal of Sexual Medicine* 6, 3111-3124 (2009).

18. Riley A, Riley E. Behavioural and clinical findings in couples where the man presents with erectile dysfunction: a retrospective study. *International Journal of Clinical Practice* 54, 220-224 (2000).

19. Hongjiun Li, Gao T, Wang R. The role of the sexual partner in managing erectile dysfunction 2016; 13, *168–Nature Reviews Urology*, 168-177.

20. Riley A. The role of the partner in erectile dysfunction and its treatment. *International Journal of Impotence Research* 2002;Suppl 1, S105-S109, DOI: 10.1038/sj/ijir/3900800.

21. Whittman D et al. Exploring the role of the partner in couples sexual recovery after surgery for prostate cancer. *Support Care Cancer* 22, 2509-2515 (2014).

22. Riley A, Riley E. Behavioural and clinical findings in couples where the man presents with erectile dysfunction: a retrospective study. *International Journal of Clinical Practice* 54, 220-224 (2000).

23. Riley A. The role of the partner in erectile dysfunction and its treatment. *International Journal of Impotence Research* 2002;Suppl 1, S105-S109, DOI: 10.1038/sj/ijir/3900800.

24. Ibid.

25. Ibid.

26. Hongjiun Li, Gao T, Wang R. The role of the sexual partner in managing erectile dysfunction 2016; 13, 168-*Nature Reviews Urology,* 168-177.

Resources

A list of websites and organizations to help couples with Erectile Dysfunction.

As a couple, you and your partner may want to continue to keep abreast of the latest research on erectile dysfunction and related conditions. Looking for additional information should not take up a great deal of time. There are creditable resources including clinics, organizations and reading material that are easily accessible. The following is a short list of resources that you and your partner may want to share between yourselves or with other couples. Each organization has a brief description, and means to access. All reading materials can be accessed through Amazon.com.

American Prostate Society
(410) 859-3735
www.americanprostatesociety.com
American Prostate Society provides support services for patients and family members affected by prostate cancer. The society provides up-to-date information on benign and malignant disorders as well.

American Urological Association (AUA)

The AUA is the leading advocate for the specialty of urology and provides invaluable support to the urologic community. The mission of AUA is to promote the highest standards of urological clinical care through education, research and the formulation of health care policy.

The Brady Urological Institute

(410) 955-6707

www.prostate.urol.jhu.edu

This organization is comprised of a group of dedicated physicians, scientists, and researchers in the Department of Urology at the Johns Hopkins Hospital whose mission is to develop and deliver excellent clinical treatment and care for urological diseases. The Web site has many articles about the latest research in prostate cancer performed at Johns Hopkins.

CIACT, Inc.

The Center for Intimacy After Cancer Therapy

301.983.9702

www.CIACT.org

Ralph and Barbara Alterowitz

P.O. Box 341388

Bethesda, Maryland 20827-1388

The Center for Intimacy after Cancer Therapy, Inc.., a 501(c)(3) nonprofit organization, is the only organization dedicated to helping couples renew their intimacy after cancer. Founders and Co-Executive Directors: Ralph and Barbara Alterowitz Ralph and Barbara are sexuality counselors certified by the American

Association of Sexuality Educators, Counselors and Therapists (AASECT), and founders of the Center for Intimacy After Cancer Therapy, Inc. (CIACT, Inc.) They frequently speak at cancer support groups and conferences, and they educate patients and the medical community on dealing with the sexual effects of cancer treatments. They provide counseling in person and via telephone or Skype. Barbara and Ralph have been happily married for over 30 years, including 20+ years "post-cancer". They walk the talk.

The James Buchanan Brady Urological Institute

The Johns Hopkins Hospital
600 North Wolfe Street
Baltimore, Maryland
http://urology.jhu.edu/

The James Buchanan Brady Urological Institute continues to strive to remain the world's leader in urology by delivering the finest patient care that includes prevention, early detection, effective treatment of localized disease, and better ways to contain advanced disease. Researchers at the Institution are committed to discovering the genes that cause debilitating urological problems in men and women as well as children.

Mayo Clinic

www.mayoclinic.org

Mayo Clinic specialists provide personalized and comprehensive care to those with erectile dysfunction. At Mayo Clinic, specialists from endocrinology, cardiovascular medicine, neurology, urology, and psychiatry and psychology work together as a multidisciplinary team to evaluate and treat each individual. This means that you're not getting just one opinion — you benefit from the knowledge and experience of each specialist. The Mayo Clinic Health System has dozens of locations in several states. Each location has its own contact number.

The Prostate Cancer Foundation
1-(800) 757-2873
www.prostatecancerfoundation.org

This foundation is the world's largest source of philanthropic support for prostate cancer research. Its primary mission is to find promising research into better treatments and a cure for prostate cancer.

US TOO
202-463-9455
Zerocancer.org
Zero-the end of Prostate Cancer
515 King Street, Suite 420
Alexandra, Virginia. 22314
info@zerocancer.org.

ZERO-the End of Prostate Cancer is the leading national nonprofit with the mission to end prostate cancer and help all who are impacted. This organization provides mentorship and counseling support services for prostate cancer patients, caregivers, and family members affected by the disease. Listed are virtual and live opportunities for interested community members to get involved in creating awareness about prostate cancer as well as opportunities to meet the top notch minds in the medical field answering your questions about prostate cancer research breakthroughs, emerging treatments, early detection, and managing your health after diagnosis.

Learn about everything from side effects of treatment, to mental health and anxiety management, to the impacts of racial disparities, and maximizing your health while living with or caring for someone who has prostate cancer.

Further Readings

100 Questions & Answers About Prostate Cancer, Second Edition
Pamela Ellsworth, MD,
Jones and Bartlett Publishing, 2009

Dr. Pamela Ellsworth addresses questions, concerns, and worries of men with prostate cancer, of their family members, and of their friends. Her goal is to help individuals feel more comfortable with the process of diagnosing prostate cancer, the treatment options for prostate cancer, and the resulting quality of life issues.

100 Questions and Answers About Prostate Disease
Kevin R. Loughlin, MD, and John Nimmo
Jones and Bartlett Publishers, 2007

According to Dr. Loughlin, benign prostate hypertrophy (BPH) is the most common benign disease of older men. Almost all men will be faced with some prostatic condition during their lifetime. The purpose of this book is to enhance understanding of the very confusing subject of prostate disease.

Prostate Cancer Survivors Speak Their Minds: Advice, Treatments, and Aftereffects
Arthur L. Burnett II and Norman S. Morris
Wiley Publisher, 2010

Personal stories show how to make the right decisions for themselves.

The Ultimate Gide on Erectile Dysfunction: Erectile Dysfunction Handbook:
The Comprehensive and essential guide to erectile dysfunction, symptoms, causes, treatment, and preventive measures
Juan Alan, MD
Independently published, 2022

Dr. Alan discusses the diagnosis and treatment of ED. As an alternative, the kindle ebook is available and can be read on any device with the free kindle app.

Glossary

Arousal and Erection Phase: Refers to the processing of sexual stimulation. The ultimate physical manifestation of sexual arousal is a penile erection.

Aspiration and irrigation: A procedure that used to aspirate or draw blood from the corpora cavernosa, and irrigation with dilute epinephrine solution under local anesthesia.

Benign prostate hyperplasia: also referred to as benign prostate enlargement. A noncancerous enlargement of the prostate.

Biopsy: A procedure in which cells are collected for microscopic examination.

Bone scan: An x-ray that looks for signs of metastasis.

Buried penis: A condition that occurs when skin and fat from the scrotum, abdomen, or thigh bury the penis, making it less visible despite it not being unusual in size.

Cavernous nerve: Nerves responsible for penile erection.

Chemotherapy: The use of chemical agents (drugs) to systematically treat cancer.

Comorbidity: A disease that is simultaneously present with another or other diseases in a patient.

Digital rectal exam: An assessment of whether a tumor is palpable by inserting a finger into the rectum.

Erect: A hardening of the penis that occurs when sponge-like tissue inside the penis fills up with blood.

Erectile dysfunction: The inability to achieve erection.

Extracorporeal shock wave therapy: Low-high intensity shock waves on the cavernosal tissue aimed at restoring or improving erectile function.

Flaccid: A penis lacking firmness.

Glans: The head or tip of the penis.

Gleason scale: A commonly used method to classify how cells appear in cancerous tissue; the less the cancerous cells look like normal cells, the more malignant the cancer; two numbers, each from 1 to 5, are assigned to the two most predominant types of cells present. These two numbers are added together to produce a Gleason score. Higher numbers indicate more aggressive cancers.

Human sexual response: A four-stage model of physiological responses to sexual stimulation.

Lymph nodes: Tissue in the lymphatic system that filter lymph fluid and help the immune system fight disease.

Malignant: Cancerous; growing rapidly and out of control.

Metastasis: Deposits of prostate cancer outside of the prostate lymph nodes.

Nocturnal erection: Referred to a nocturnal penile tumescence. A spontaneous erection of the penis during sleep or when awaking up

Non-Invasive: A medical procedure not requiring the introduction of instruments into the body.

Orgasm and ejaculation phase: The perception of pleasurable sensations with sexual climax. Ejaculation is the physical response to the message.

Oncologist: A medical doctor qualified to diagnose and treat tumors.

Penile vascular surgery: A surgical process of connecting inferior penile veins are arteries to improve or treat erectile dysfunction.

Peyronie's disease: A penile disorder that causes the penis to bend caused either by scar tissue, plaque, hard lumps, or some other build up creates an abnormal penile curvature.

Platelet-rich plasma: Blood that consists of plasma and blood cells that play an important role in healing throughout the body. Platelets contain growth factors that can trigger cell reproduction and tissue regeneration of healing in the treated area.

Platcau phase: The second phase of the sexual response cycle in which breathing becomes more rapid and muscles continue to tense.

Priapism: Painful prolonged erection of the penis, without sexual arousal.

Prostate biopsy: Diagnostic technique for prostate cancer in which a needle instrument is used to sample multiple prostate pieces (usually 12) for pathological assessment.

Prostate cancer: The presence of malignant cells in the prostate. .

Prostate-specific antigen (PSA) Test: Blood test used to screen for prostate cancer. Measures the amount of prostate-specific antigen (PSA) in the blood.

Prostate-specific antigen: A protein produced by cancerous and noncancerous tissue in the prostate.

Prostate: A small gland that sits below the bladder in males.

Priapism: A unwanted, persistent erection. It may occur spontaneously or from certain antidepressants or erectile dysfunction drugs.

Prostate specific antigen (PSA): A chemical produced by benign and cancerous prostate tissue. The levels seem to be higher with prostate cancer.

Pudendal; nerve: A major nerve in the pelvic region that sends motor and sensation information to the genital area.

Risk factor: A condition or behavior that increases the chance of developing a disease.

Radical prostatectomy: Surgical removal of the entire prostate

Resolution phase: A gradual return to the resting state that may take several hours.

Sex hormone binding globin (SHBG) Test: A test used to detect level of testosterone production.

Sexual desire and libido phase: Refers to sexual interest and the motivation to seek sexual arousal.

Seminal vesicles: Either of a pair of pouch like glands situated on each side of the male urinary bladder that secrete seminal fluid and nourish and promote the movement of spermatozoa through the urethra.

Sickle cell: A heredity form of anemia in which a mutated form of hemoglobin distorts the red blood cells into a crescent or sickle-shape. These cells do not bend or move easily and can block blood flow to the rest of the body, including the pelvic region.

Side effects: Problems that occur in addition to the desired therapeutic effect.

Stem cell therapy: A transplant procedure used to regenerate or replace cells damaged by disease or chemotherapy.

Testosterone: A male hormone.

Urinary control: Ability to control the voiding of urine.

Vasocogention: Increased blood flow that causes swelling in the genitals.

Venous leak: A type of sexual dysfunction where men experience venous leaks in the penile tissue causing soft erection.

Index

About the Author

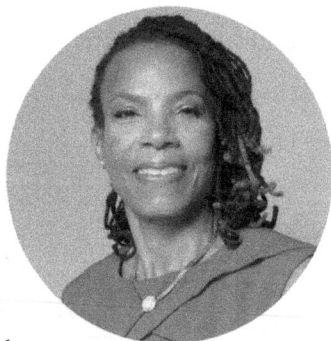

Elisha J. Nixon Cobb, Ph.D, M.Ed. is a retired Associate Professor in health education, public speaker, and health coach. She is CEO and founder of Midlife Strong, LLC., an educational organization, where she teaches midlife individuals over age 40 years how to live longer healthier lives through education and health promotion. Her dissertation on menopause in African American rural women and her course on menopause prepares women of color to embrace their bodily changes as a well-deserved rite of passage.

After earning her master's and PhD degrees in health education from The Pennsylvania State University in State College, Pennsylvania, she worked in The Multicultural Resource Center as a academic counselor for students of color. She then became Assistant Dean of Studies at Lafayette College in Easton, Pennsylvania. Dr. Nixon moved on to become tenured faculty at Kean University in New Jersey and part-time instructor at Alvernia University in Pennsylvania.

Dr. Nixon has written several books and articles on the subject of menopause, and how to improve students' critical thinking on health issues related to behavior change. She has also provided counseling support services to families on a myriad of behavioral health-related concerns. On the basis of her background in health education and counseling, and her experience coping with her husband's struggle with erectile dysfunction, she has extended her counseling services to include providing support to family members impacted by the disease, with a special focus on men and their partners dealing with erectile dysfunction.

9 781736 880333